Cortisol - Beyond a Simple Hormone

Edited by Diana Loreta Păun

Published in London, United Kingdom

Cortisol - Beyond a Simple Hormone
http://dx.doi.org/10.5772/intechopen.1008660
Edited by Diana Loreta Păun

Contributors
Abdulrahman G. Alharbi, Ali M. Alalawi, Bandar D. Alrehaili, Bandar D. Alrehaili, Cristina Criveanu, Daniela Greere, Diana Loreta Păun, Esha Elizabeth Cherian, Jubbin Jagan Jacob, Mohammed H. Alsubhi, Tahani A. Saeedi

First published in London, United Kingdom, 2026 by IntechOpen
IntechOpen is the global imprint of INTECHOPEN LIMITED, registered in England and Wales, registration number: 11086078, 167-169 Great Portland Street, London, W1W 5PF, United Kingdom

For EU product safety concerns: IN TECH d.o.o., Prolaz Marije Krucifikse Kozulić 3, 51000 Rijeka, Croatia, info@intechopen.com or visit our website at intechopen.com.

British Library Cataloguing-in-Publication Data
A catalogue record for this book is available from the British Library

Cortisol - Beyond a Simple Hormone
Edited by Diana Loreta Păun
p. cm.
Print ISBN 978-1-83635-241-9
Online ISBN 978-1-83635-240-2
eBook (PDF) ISBN 978-1-83635-242-6

If disposing of this product, please recycle the paper responsibly.

Meet the editor

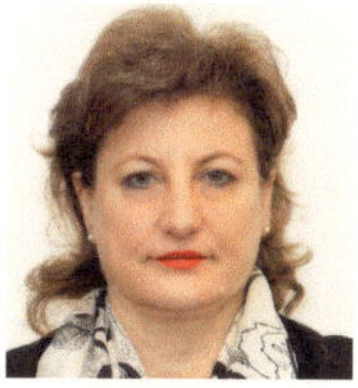

Diana Loreta Păun, MD, Ph.D., FACE, is Professor of Endocrinology at the University of Medicine and Pharmacy and an endocrinologist at Bucharest University Emergency Hospital, Bucharest, Romania. Dr. Păun has acquired a comprehensive array of qualifications within her field, encompassing Diabetology, Osteoporosis, Endocrine Ultrasonography, and Public Health. She was General Manager of the CI Parhon National Institute of Endocrinology from 2006 to 2015. Furthermore, between 2015 and 2026, she served as the Presidential Advisor for Health to the President of Romania. Dr. Păun is a Fellow of the American College of Endocrinology and former President of the Romanian Chapter of the American Association of Clinical Endocrinologists (AACE), member of the Romanian Society of Endocrinology, of Psihoneuroendocrinology, and the Romanian Associations of Clinical Endocrinologists.

Contents

Preface **IX**

Section 1
General Aspects of Cortisol Biology **1**

Chapter 1 3
Introductory Chapter: Cortisol – An Intelligent Regulator of Physiological Balance
by Diana Loreta Păun

Chapter 2 7
Cortisol: Transport
by Bandar D. Alrehaili, Tahani A. Saeedi, Mohammed H. Alsubhi and Ali M. Alalawi

Chapter 3 23
Cortisol: Metabolism
by Abdulrahman G. Alharbi and Bandar D. Alrehaili

Section 2
HPA Axis Testing and Corticosteroid Therapy in Clinical Practice **41**

Chapter 4 43
Laboratory Evaluation of the Hypothalamic-Pituitary-Adrenal Axis
by Daniela Greere and Diana Loreta Păun

Chapter 5 65
Adrenal Insufficiency Associated with Inhaled Corticosteroid Use
by Esha Elizabeth Cherian and Jubbin Jagan Jacob

Chapter 6 87
Corticosteroid Therapy in Rheumatology: Essential Treatment, Challenges and Solutions
by Cristina Criveanu

Preface

In an era of digitalization and artificial intelligence, a book addressing a hormone of survival and adaptation to stress represents an ambitious endeavor, yet one of practical importance for physicians across different specialties.

Cortisol remains a remarkable hormone, both for its effects on the organism and for its use in the treatment of various diseases, including cancer therapy.

This book aims to provide an exploration of the intricate mechanisms of cortisol secretion, transport and distribution, metabolism, regulation, and actions, while also broadening its scope by emphasizing the therapeutic benefits of steroids through an analysis of corticosteroid therapy from the perspective of balancing beneficial effects against adverse reactions. Future pharmacological strategies will further enhance therapeutic benefits while reducing the complications associated with such therapy.

The book extensively explains the cellular mechanisms of cortisol action and reviews and analyzes their clinical implications. By way of example, the circadian pattern of cortisol secretion reveals a crucial homeostatic mechanism that optimizes functions associated with metabolism, cognition, and immunity.

We wish the reader enthusiasm in exploring the mysteries of cortisol, this intelligent hormone, and aim to provide, in an accessible format, the major advances achieved in understanding its mechanisms of action and the pathology associated with this fascinating hormone.

I want to express my gratitude to IntechOpen, to the authors of the chapters who chose to support me in this endeavor, and to extend my thanks and deepest appreciation to Ms. Iva Horvat, Publishing Process Manager, for her patience and availability throughout the preparation of this book. I am equally grateful to my patients, as well as to my students and residents, who continue to inspire me and to whom I especially dedicate this book.

Diana Loreta Păun
Department of Endocrinology,
"Carol Davila" University of Medicine and Pharmacy,
Bucharest, Romania

Section 1

General Aspects of Cortisol Biology

Chapter 1

Introductory Chapter: Cortisol – An Intelligent Regulator of Physiological Balance

Diana Loreta Păun

1. Introduction

Within the complex ensemble of the human hormonal system, cortisol stands out as the most remarkable hormone. It is essential for survival, as its absence from the body for more than 24 hours is synonymous with death. At the same time, cortisol is the principal hormone responsible for adaptation to stress, with its secretion increasing dramatically under stressful conditions. Cortisol also regulates our daily activity according to the light-dark or sleep-wake cycle. Moreover, it is the foundation of the most frequently used medical therapy—corticosteroid treatment.

All these arguments, which demonstrate cortisol's role as a regulator of the body's homeostatic balance, justify dedicating a book to this remarkable hormone—one intended to be only a small drop in an ocean of the unknown. Furthermore, we learn about cortisol, the more unanswered questions emerge. This book proposes an exploration of the physiology of this hormone, aiming to present the current state of knowledge in the field while also offering new perspectives with therapeutic implications.

2. From history to everyday-life adaptation

First isolated from adrenal extracts by Calvin Kendall in 1946, alongside three other steroid compounds [1], cortisol was central to the awarding of the 1950 Nobel Prize in Physiology or Medicine to three researchers (Edward Calvin Kendall, Tadeus Reichstein, and Philip Showalter Hench). Beyond elucidating its chemical structure, the biological effects of the hormone were demonstrated, forming the basis for the use of cortisone in the treatment of rheumatoid arthritis [2]. This discovery represented a pioneering moment in therapy, demonstrating for the first time the anti-inflammatory effects of cortisone and having a major impact on the treatment of inflammatory, allergic, and autoimmune diseases. It laid the foundation for the modern development of corticosteroids in medicine.

Of particular importance is the regulation of cortisol secretion, which is ensured by the hypothalamic-pituitary–adrenal (HPA) axis, both under basal conditions and in response to stress. ACTH is the main hormone stimulating cortisol secretion and is itself stimulated by corticotropin-releasing hormone (CRH) and arginine vasopressin (AVP), produced by the paraventricular nucleus (PVN) of the hypothalamus.

CRH and AVP bind to specific receptors, CRH-R1 and V1B, at the level of the anterior pituitary, inducing the release of adrenocorticotropic hormone (ACTH) into the circulation. ACTH exerts trophic effects on the adrenal cortex and stimulates the secretion of cortisol and adrenal androgens from the fasciculata and reticularis zones of the adrenal cortex [3].

The principal mechanism for maintaining normal plasma cortisol concentrations is negative feedback inhibition exerted by cortisol on the secretion of ACTH and CRH.

Under basal conditions, cortisol is secreted in a circadian and ultradian rhythm, with a peak around 8:00 a.m. The circadian rhythm of cortisol secretion is determined by episodic hormone release controlled by the central nervous system, which regulates both the frequency and amplitude of secretory episodes of CRH and ACTH. Cortisol levels are lowest in the late evening hours and continue to decline during the early hours of sleep, potentially becoming undetectable in plasma. Between the third and fifth hours of sleep, an increase in secretion occurs; however, major secretory episodes begin between the sixth and eighth hours of sleep, reach a peak, and then gradually decline upon awakening. Approximately half of daily cortisol production occurs during this interval. Throughout the day, secretion decreases progressively. The circadian rhythm may be disrupted by changes in light exposure, alterations in meal timing, and pathological conditions such as physical or psychological stress, disorders of the central nervous system and pituitary gland, Cushing's syndrome, liver disease, chronic renal failure, or alcoholism.

ACTH and cortisol levels rise within minutes after the onset of a stressor, such as surgery or hypoglycemic episodes. If stress is prolonged, this response suppresses the circadian rhythm.

3. Without cortisol, there is no life

The impact of cortisol on the body is essential, as this hormone plays a fundamental role in survival. It is also a key hormone in the stress response. Its major biological effects are metabolic in nature and act on carbohydrate, lipid, and protein metabolism [4]. Cortisol primarily exerts a catabolic effect, promoting the mobilization of energy reserves, which is essential for adaptation to stress.

However, cortisol is more than a simple hormone, due to its anti-inflammatory, antiallergic, and immunosuppressive roles in the body. These functions have particular significance, forming the basis for the widespread use of cortisol derivatives as medication across a broad range of pathologies [5].

4. Future perspectives

Cortisol plays an extremely important role in all physiological processes of the body, from growth and sexual development to the regulation of metabolism and the stress response.

The intricate mechanisms regulating the secretion of this hormone—mechanisms that adapt to the circadian rhythm and are modulated by stress—require deeper understanding, and any new scientific approach to this hormone may shed further light on its complexity.

In the era of digitalization and artificial intelligence, we must understand the lessons offered by cortisol—this intelligent hormone. New therapeutic strategies based on the physiological secretory profile of cortisol, or novel markers of response to corticosteroid therapy, could enable personalized management and improve the quality of life of patients undergoing corticosteroid treatment.

Acknowledgements

The author acknowledges the use of ChatGPT for language polishing of the manuscript.

Author details

Diana Loreta Păun
Department of Endocrinology, "Carol Davila" University of Medicine and Pharmacy, Bucharest, Romania

*Address all correspondence to: dianaloreta_paun@yahoo.com

References

[1] Simoni RD, Hill RL, Vaughan M. The isolation of thyroxine and cortisone: The work of Edward C. Kendall. The Journal of Biological Chemistry. 2002;**277**(21):e10

[2] Hench PS, Kendall EC, Slocumb CH, Polley HF. The effect of a hormone of the adrenal cortex (17-hydroxy-11-dehydrocorticosterone; compound E) and of pituitary adrenocorticotropic hormone on rheumatoid arthritis. Proceedings of the Staff Meetings. Mayo Clinic. 1949;**24**:181-197

[3] Spiga F, Walker JJ, Terry JR, Lightman SL. HPA axis-rhythms. Comprehensive Physiology. 2014;**4**: 1273-1298. DOI: 10.1002/cphy.c140003

[4] Timmermans S, Souffriau J, Libert C. A general introduction to glucocorticoid biology. Frontiers in Immunology. 2019;**10**:1-17

[5] Coutinho AE, Chapman KE. The anti-inflammatory and immunosuppressive effects of glucocorticoids, recent developments and mechanistic insights. Molecular and Cellular Endocrinology. 2011;**335**(1):2-13

Chapter 2

Cortisol: Transport

Bandar D. Alrehaili, Tahani A. Saeedi, Mohammed H. Alsubhi and Ali M. Alalawi

Abstract

Cortisol is a glucocorticoid hormone and is synthesized in the middle layer of adrenal cortex in response to adrenocorticotropic hormone. It has importance in metabolism, homeostasis, and physiological stress management. This chapter focuses on cortisol transport pathways, including corticosteroid-binding globulin and albumin, ensuring appropriate hormone distribution. It will also provide a comprehensive review of cortisol receptors functions, genomic and non-genomic signaling pathways, and related mechanisms that facilitate the biological effects of cortisol in various tissues. Mechanisms of glucocorticoid receptors and cortisol tissue-specific access and distribution will be discussed in detail. The purposes of cortisol-binding protein dynamics and tissue-specific distribution patterns that determine cortisol bioavailability and target tissue exposure will be described. The advanced knowledge of cortisol transport would light new directions toward improving new therapeutic approaches for endocrine-related diseases.

Keywords: cortisol, glucocorticoid receptors, corticosteroid, albumin, globulin

1. Introduction

1.1 Background of cortisol

Glucocorticoids are hormones, and their excretions are regulated by hypothalamic and hypophyseal hormones. Using the abbreviation "Cort" that refers to cortisol or corticosteroids as a synonym of stress is common and not precise. Scientists should not use stress hormones to refer to glucocorticoids because their response to a stressor is not a primary function of glucocorticoids [1]. Corticotropin-releasing hormone (CRH) normally has negative correlation with cortisol blood level. The stimulation of secretion of CRH into the portal circulation leads to the activation of the anterior pituitary to secrete adrenocorticotropic hormone (ACTH) into the systemic circulation. ACTH is carried into the adrenal cortex, which causes the secretion of cortisol into the circulation [2]. The blood level of cortisol acts as a signal to regulate cortisol secretion by negative feedback mechanism at the pituitary, hypothalamus, and hippocampus [3]. Dysregulation in cortisol secretion is associated with cortisol-related comorbidities. Mild autonomous cortisol secretion is one of the most common hormonal irregularities in patients with adrenal gland tumor [4]. Elevated cortisol levels are associated with psychiatric illnesses such as depression and anxiety.

They also affect memory, coordination, and emotional constancy [5]. In normal conditions, cortisol is secreted under circadian regulation and any disruptions in this diurnal rhythm cause adverse health outcomes, including high risk of inflammation, infection, and cancer [6]. The cortisol transport that repeats the right diurnal slope offers further metabolic benefits, such as adjusted body weight, blood glucose, and vascular pressure [7]. The hypothalamic-pituitary-adrenal (HPA) axis is a neuroendocrine system that links the brain with the periphery of the body. Cortisol is the final product of the HPA axis during acute disorders in humans [8, 9]. Feedback mechanism plays a critical role in maintaining normal cortisol levels in the circulation. The negative feedback mechanism limits the activation of HPA axis when cortisol sends signals by glucocorticoid receptor (GR) binding in peripheral tissues. These signals inhibit ACTH expression, reducing brain capacity to initiate the HPA axis [10]. This system ensures that an optimum level of cortisol is available in peripheral tissues, indicating the importance of cortisol's biological effects. Glucocorticoids are involved in the regulation of immunity, metabolic pathways, reproductive system, behavior, and cognitive functions [11].

1.2 Chapter scope and objectives

The goal of this chapter is to provide booklovers with an advanced knowledge of cortisol transport, covering molecular pathways and clinical purposes. This chapter will provide an overview of the biology of cortisol, beginning with its hormonal regulation, endocrine synthesis, circulatory transport, cellular mechanisms, and clearance pathways. Here are three main objectives of this chapter:

Primary goals:

1. *Describe transport and distribution mechanisms*: Elucidate the function of binding proteins, free *versus* bound hormone dynamics, and tissue-specific distribution patterns that determine cortisol bioavailability and target tissue exposure.

2. *Explain cellular mechanisms of action*: Explain the role of the glucocorticoid receptor, genomic and non-genomic signaling pathways, and intracellular mechanisms that mediate cortisol's diverse biological effects.

3. *Review and interpret clinical implications*: Emphasize on the pathophysiology of cortisol transport-related disorders, including hypo- and hypercortisolism, and review current and developing new medications.

By the end of this chapter, readers will have a thorough understanding of cortisol transport, allowing them to better understand its physiological circulation, identify pathological variations related to cortisol transport, and realize the importance of an advanced understanding of cortisol transport to improve therapeutic approaches.

1.3 Circadian rhythm of cortisol production

Secretion of cortisol in living things shows a unique and well-preserved 24-hour rhythm, which reflects the importance of time-based hormone regulation. Under normal conditions, the cortisol blood level is usually low or undetectable in the blood at midnight, which progressively increases to reach a peak in the early morning, after which the cortisol level gradually falls during the daytime until reaching its lowest level at midnight [7, 12]. Cortisol's circadian rhythm also reflects chronological regulation of the HPA axis, with the highest cortisol blood concentrations in the early morning and the lowest at midnight [13]. The suprachiasmatic nucleus (SCN) of the hypothalamus works as the main circadian clock, organizing CRH release that energizes rhythmic ACTH production [13, 14].

Cortisol's circadian rhythm helps in preparing the body for anticipated metabolic desires related to daily activity arrangements. Cortisol blood level normally rises throughout the last part of sleep time until reaching its peak level nearly 30 minutes after awakening, known as the cortisol awakening response (CAR) [15, 16]. During the day, cortisol level is progressively reduced until reaching its nadir level at midnight. This chronological pattern is complexly related to sleep manner. So, the secretion of cortisol is decreased in slow-wave sleep (SWS) and increased in rapid eye-movement (REM) sleep and upon awakening [17, 18].

This circadian pattern denotes a crucial homeostatic mechanism that optimizes functions associated with metabolism, cognition, and immunity. Modifications in cortisol's circadian rhythm cause pathological outcomes in essential physiological processes, such as glucose metabolism, immune system function, memory, coordination, emotional regulation, acute coronary syndrome, arrhythmias, and stroke [7, 19, 20]. The association between the circadian rhythm and an individual's daily life is obvious, especially for people who are involved in a whole day or night shift work [21]. They have changes in the cortisol production pattern to adjust to the modified sleep-wake transition rather than following cortisol's circadian rhythm [22].

Using cortisol's circadian rhythm as a diagnostic tool has become noticeable in evaluating a cortisol-related disorder, such as Cushing's syndrome where disturbance of the diurnal rhythm causes its fundamental feature [23, 24]. A highly specific and sensitive diagnostic technique in diagnosing Cushing syndrome is known as late night salivary cortisol (LNSC) [25]. This method senses abnormal elevation of cortisol level during the physiological cortisol nadir level, which is considered as an initial marker of autonomous cortisol secretion.

Nevertheless, many influences can affect the cortisol production pattern, such as differences in age and body weight, degree of stress and inflammation, and psychiatric and sleep disorders. Briefly, an elevation of evening cortisol levels may be caused by acute psychological stress, which creates diagnostic difficulties when comparing physiological and pathological states. For example, obstructive sleep apnea syndrome (OSAS) has been associated with reduced morning salivary cortisol levels that form a pseudo-Cushing's state leading to vague endocranial evaluation [26].

2. Transport and distribution

Subsequent to cortisol synthesis and circadian regulation, it must be transported from blood circulation to target tissues to apply its biological effects. This complicated distribution system ensures that cortisol reaches its target spots and keeps appropriate hormone concentration for ideal physiological role.

2.1 Binding proteins

Secretion of cortisol from the adrenal gland into circulation is usually in forms bound to specific plasma proteins, such as corticosteroid-binding globulin (CBG) and albumin. The bound complex of cortisol and CBG is distributed in a 1:1 ratio that modulates the release of cortisol across the tissues. So, the percentage of free form of the cortisol is directly related to the cortisol-CBG complex, which is determined by two factors: binding affinity and its concentration [27]. A minor amount (3–5%) of circulating cortisol is in unbound bioactive form, a lipophilic form that enables cortisol to translocate from capillaries to tissues primarily *via* passive diffusion and attach to its targeted receptors (**Figure 1**) [23]. This cortisol-receptor complex plays different vital roles, such as metabolism regulation, immune response, cardiovascular function, and stress acclimatization.

Figure 1 shows the estimated percentages of cortisol bound forms and free cortisol in human blood. Over 80% of total cortisol is bound to corticosteroid-binding globulin, and around 14% of total cortisol is bound to albumin. The unbound form of cortisol represents 3–5% of total plasma cortisol in human blood.

2.1.1 Corticosteroid-binding globulin (CBG)

A major amount of total circulating cortisol is bound to CBG. This plasma protein has a high affinity for cortisol, and each CBG molecule has a specific steroid-binding site. CBG controls the bioavailability and metabolic clearance of glucocorticoids [23]. The high-affinity form of CBG works as a safeguard for cortisol to be available in plasma for distribution to target cells and to prevent cortisol degradation during delivery (**Table 1**). In other words, it aids as the major transport glycoprotein for cortisol, and over 80% of total plasma-bound cortisol binds to CBG (**Figure 1**) [23, 32]. CBG was discovered in 1950, it belongs to the serine protease inhibitor (SERPIN) family and is known as transcortin [33]. It is a 50 to 60 kDa glycoprotein that acts as the primarily carrier for glucocorticoids such as cortisol. CBG is a polypeptide of about 383 amino acid residues secreted from liver cells. This polypeptide is secreted after its cleavage from 22 amino acid peptides and is monomeric, which means that each molecule has one steroid-binding site that circulates in the body at the concentration of 175 to 365 nmol/L [27, 34]. Saturated plasma concentrations of CBG are 450–600 nmol/L in healthy individuals. Glucocorticoid delivery occurs *via* cleavage of the reactive center loop of CBG by neutrophil elastase resulting in irreversible conversion to a low-affinity form to release cortisol [35]. The transport of cortisol

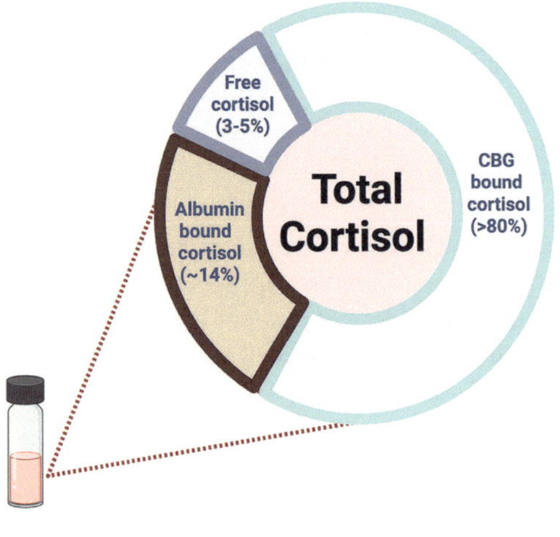

Figure 1.
Cortisol distribution in the blood.

Cortisol forms Parameters	Bound cortisol		Free cortisol
	CBG	Albumin	
Bioactivity	*No*	*No*	*Yes* [28]
Binding affinity	*High* [29]	*Low* [29]	—
CM penetration	*No* [28]	*No* [28]	*Yes* [28]
BBB penetration	*No* [30]	*Yes* [30]	*Limited* [31]

The above table shows some properties of bound cortisol and unbound cortisol that affect cortisol distribution in peripheral tissues. Abbreviations: CBG: corticosteroid-binding globulin; CM: cell membrane; BBB: blood-brain barrier.

Table 1.
Biological and pharmacokinetic properties of cortisol forms.

is mediated through two additional mechanisms: acidosis and pyrexia. The cortisol binding is reversibly attenuated by acidosis and pyrexia, whereas it is irreversibly reduced by neutrophil elastase, which converts it into a low-affinity form observed in conditions like sepsis (**Figure 2**) [34]. Thus, CBG plays a crucial role in inflammation, as defects in cortisol transport can increase the mortality rate.

2.1.2 Albumin

Albumin is the second transporter for cortisol in the circulation, and around 14% of total plasma-bound cortisol is bound to it (**Figure 1**) [32]. Unlike CBG, albumin shows low-affinity binding to cortisol (**Table 1**) [29], allowing bioavailability of the bound cortisol for discharge. This low-affinity binding form stabilizes availability of the cortisol-bound form as an additional transport capacity, when CBG-bound cortisol is reduced because of abnormal circumstances. So, the importance of albumin-bound cortisol has become evident under CBG synthesis-related diseases including hepatic disorders or the presence of CBG competitive agents at CBG-binding sites. Albumin serves as a substitute carrier protein to ensure cortisol distribution despite potential disruptions in the major cortisol carrier protein to maintain necessary cortisol actions [36].

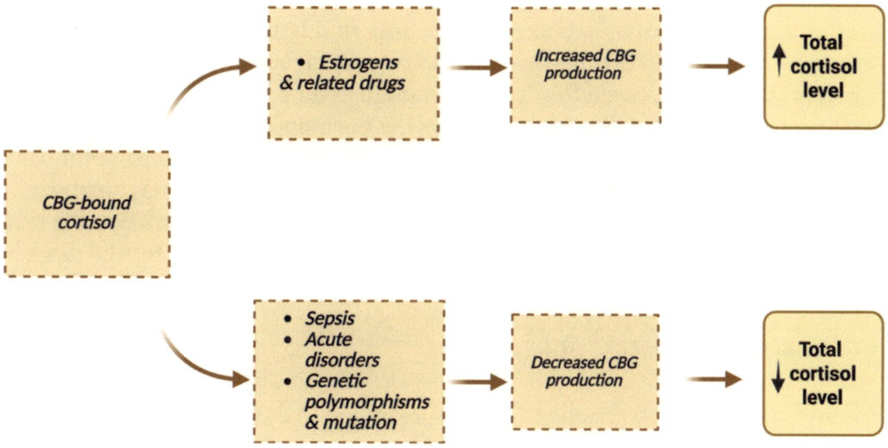

Figure 2.
Factors affecting CBG production.

2.1.3 Transport dynamics

The cortisol-binding proteins create a dynamic equilibrium that modifies physiological demands to ensure persistence of critical cortisol activity. Differences in concentrations of carrier proteins and environmental conditions, including pH, temperature, and the presence of competitive agents at protein-binding sites of cortisol, can change this steadiness, affecting the amount of bound cortisol and free cortisol. This dynamic equilibrium system allows rapid changes in free cortisol bioavailability in response to altering physiological situations (*more detail in Section 2.2.2*).

2.2 Free vs. bound cortisol

The dissimilarity between the two forms of circulating cortisol expresses the movement of cortisol between plasma and tissues. Metabolism and excretion of cortisol rely on the presence and absence of plasma proteins. Both free and bound forms of cortisol are transported to the extracellular compartment. The free form of cortisol passes easily through the cellular wall to attach to its targeted receptors and is considered as biologically active form [37, 38]. The release of the active form of cortisol follows the law of mass action. This highlights the significance of the bound protein, as any modifications in the affinity and concentration can affect the physiological activity of the free form of cortisol. The concentration of free cortisol may change depending upon its secretion from the adrenal cortex, which could lead to disproportionately increased quantity [27]. The bound form of cortisol works as a tank, which is a critical job when fast cortisol movement is required or during specific conditions such as stress periods. The protein-bound form of cortisol can be rapidly liberated from its carrier protein to meet the physiological requests. Thus, this binding system creates a balanced mechanism that ensures steady hormone levels even though there are variations in production or excretion rates (**Table 1**).

2.2.1 The free hormone hypothesis

The free hormone hypothesis claims that only the unbound fraction of the circulating hormone is able to pass through the cell membrane and exert its influences. Examples of free fraction hormones include cortisol, thyroid hormones, sex hormones, and vitamin D metabolites. These unbound hormones are hydrophobic and expected to passively diffuse through the plasma membrane. However, the free hormone is not the sole reason for the hormones to enter cells. The movement of free fraction is affected by the dissociation of the hormone from its plasma-binding protein, the rate of blood flow, the rate of cellular uptake, and catabolism of hormone within its target cell. These represent components of the free hormone transport process as called by Mendel. The concentration of the free hormone affects the transport process into the cell when the transport rate is not rate-limiting for the targeted cell [39, 40].

2.2.2 Dynamic equilibrium of cortisol

Bound and unbound fractions of cortisol continue in dynamic equilibrium. This equilibrium is affected by CBG release in response to internal and external temperatures. The binding affinity of cortisol to CBG decreases by 16-folds when the temperature raises from 35 to 42°C. Systemic inflammation by proteolysis can change the binding affinity of cortisol to its carrier proteins. Enzymes, including neutrophil elastase and 11 beta-hydroxysteroid dehydrogenase (11βHSD), can affect cortisol bioavailability for binding to its targeted receptor [28]. Other hormones and related drugs can also influence the dynamic equilibrium of cortisol. Estrogen rushes CBG synthesis from the liver; therefore, the cortisol level is regularly measured when mitotane, an estrogen-like medication, is used [29]. The increase in CBG production by oral contraceptive medications causes misinterpretation of cortisol action depending on the total cortisol level (**Figure 2**) [40–43]. However, sepsis and other acute disorders are associated with subabnormal levels of cortisol due to reduction of CBG levels and associated hypoproteinemia. Polymorphisms in the structure of cortisol-binding sites and *SERPINA6* mutations are associated with low levels or no CBG in the circulation (**Figure 2**). Patients with these genetic variations usually have normal ACTH and free cortisol levels in serum and saliva, but the total cortisol level is low or undetectable [28, 40]. This indicates the importance of assessing both total and free cortisol levels for precise diagnosis of hypoadrenalism. Exploring these factors is crucial for predicting the correct clinical manifestations and therapies.

Factors influence CBG synthesis and availability of cortisol. Estrogens and related drugs, including mitotane and oral contraceptives, induce CBG production, which results in increased total cortisol levels. However, pathological disorders such as sepsis, genetic polymorphisms, and mutations cause reduction in CBG production leading to reduced total cortisol levels.

2.2.3 Clinical significance of free cortisol

Plasma-free cortisol level offers a precise assessment of the active hormone availability in the circulation. The accuracy of measuring cortisol level is crucial in hypoadrenalism to avoid misdiagnosis and optimize the stress dose during the treatment of patients with drug-induced hypoadrenalism [28]. Quantification of plasma-free cortisol levels shows a clear association between manifestations and therapeutic outcomes. Despite the importance of free cortisol measurement, there are clinical and technical difficulties in applying it to a wide-range of clinical applications [28, 44].

2.3 Tissue distribution and access

Distribution of free cortisol into its target cells requires several mechanisms to pass various organs and cells. Conversion of cortisol from cortisone is catalyzed by 11beta-hydroxysteroid dehydrogenase type1 (βHSD1) when the cells are intact, and the enzyme activity acts as reductase. However, cortisol-cortisone conversion occurs when cells are disrupted, and the enzyme activity is dehydrogenase. This indicates tissue-specific regulation by βHSD1, which can be a therapeutic target for the treatment of patients with metabolic disorders, such as type 2 diabetes mellitus [45].

2.3.1 Mechanism of tissue access and tissue-specific distribution

The hydrophobic nature of free cortisol allows it to pass into cells through passive diffusion and move along a concentration gradient. There are several players that affect the penetration of cortisol into its targeted cells. These factors include cortisol bioavailability, concentration gradient, tissue specificity, and regional blood flow. The distribution of cortisol through body organs shows variability, which indicates tissue-specificity. The variability of cortisol distribution among different tissues has occurred because of cortisol tissue-specific activity and anatomical properties. For example, the central nervous system is associated with difficulties for cortisol penetration because of the blood-brain barrier, demanding either specific escorting pathways or high plasma cortisol levels. High concentration of cortisol in plasma has major role in diffusing cortisol into the CNS compared to transporters [31]. Tissues show different capacities for cortisol penetration depending on the blood flow and properties of cell membrane. Tissues in the liver, kidneys, and lungs have fast uptake of cortisol due to high blood flow rates. These tissues act as the main targets for cortisol's metabolic and anti-inflammatory effects and normally determine rapid balance with plasma hormone concentrations. However, tissues with low blood flow may have deferred or limited hormone access, which makes alterations in cortisol bioavailability and outcomes [46].

2.3.2 Factors affecting distribution

Many factors affect the tissue distribution of cortisol, which controls proper cortisol transport into cells. Differences in carrier protein levels can influence cortisol bioavailability in tissues under certain conditions. Specific tissues may generate their own CBG, leading to the creation of microenvironments with altered cortisol-binding capacity, while acute disorders and sepsis can decrease local CBG levels through proteolytic cleavage by neutrophil elastase [28, 40]. Tissue blood supply performs an essential function, as areas with higher blood flow have better cortisol access, while conditions that reduce blood flow, such as shock or vascular disease, can impede cortisol access to the affected tissue. Some tissues may have special transport mechanisms that may induce or inhibit cortisol penetration into cells. These mechanisms can be controlled by several influences, such as cortisol forms, pathological conditions, and medications, which add additional complexity to the distribution of cortisol into tissues [40–42].

2.3.3 Physiological implications

The cortisol distribution system helps target tissues take up optimal concentrations of cortisol for its cellular roles while preserving endocrine homeostasis. Cortisol distribution regulates refluxes to stress and required metabolic changes while maintaining tissue-specific regulation of cortisol activity. Once cortisol reaches target tissues, it must involve certain cellular mechanisms to exert its physiological effects.

3. Cellular mechanisms of action

Once cortisol passes the cell membrane, specific cellular mechanism is involved to exert the biological effects of cortisol. The signaling pathway starts with the binding of cortisol to its receptors inside the cell, leading to receptor activation and facilitating physiological influences across the body.

3.1 Glucocorticoid receptors

The NR3C1 gene codes for the glucocorticoid receptor (GR), which is a member of the nuclear receptor superfamily of ligand-activated transcription factors. These factors are responsible for the biological effects of endogenous glucocorticoids, such as cortisol, and synthetic agents such as dexamethasone and prednisolone. The GR has a modular structure that is typical of nuclear receptors. It has different functional domains that work together to recognize ligands, bind DNA, regulate transcription, and interact with coregulatory proteins. The receptor has four parts: the N-terminal domain (NTD), the DNA-binding domain (DBD), a hinge region, and the ligand-binding domain (LBD). Each of these domains helps the receptor be flexible in how it controls things and how it responds to transcription in different types of cells. The activation function-1 (AF-1) region is in the N-terminal domain. It controls ligand-independent transcriptional activation and is an important interface for bringing in transcriptional coactivators and parts of the basal transcriptional machinery. The NTD is different from other domains because it is intrinsically disordered in structure [47, 48].

The DNA-binding domain (DBD) is one of the parts of nuclear receptors that do not change much. There are two zinc-finger motifs in it that let it bind to certain sequences of glucocorticoid response elements (GREs) in the promoter or enhancer regions of target genes. The first zinc finger is mostly responsible for recognizing DNA, while the second helps receptors dimerize and stabilize DNA interactions. This domain is very important for genomic signaling because it makes sure that only certain GRE sequences bind to it, which in turn controls transcriptional specificity [49]. The hinge region is a flexible part that connects the DBD to the ligand-binding domain. It is next to the DBD. There are nuclear localization signals (NLS) in the hinge that become visible when a ligand binds. This helps the receptor move from the cytoplasm to the nucleus. This area also helps the receptor change shape and may be involved in interactions between proteins [48].

The activation function-2 (AF-2) region is in the C-terminal ligand-binding domain (LBD), which is what makes glucocorticoids bind tightly. The LBD has a hydrophobic pocket that holds steroid ligands. When a ligand binds to it, it changes shape in a way that keeps the receptor in its active state. These changes in shape help the protein break away from inhibitory chaperone complexes and allow transcriptional coactivators with LXXLL motifs, like members of the steroid receptor coactivator (SRC) family, to bind. The LBD also helps receptors dimerize, interact with corepressors, and change the amount of transcription that happens based on the type of ligand that is bound [50, 51].

3.2 Genomic effects

Glucocorticoids suppress the immune system *via* genomic pathway, and the interaction of glucocorticoid (GC) with its cytosolic receptor leads to translocation of GC-GR complex into the nucleus to activate gene transcription *via* a homodimer binding to GR element response (GRE) at the promoter of target genes [52]. This direct regulation allows recruitment of coactivator or corepressor proteins to modify chromatin structure, which inhibits the transcription of inflammatory genes, leading to the initiation of the anti-inflammatory effects [53]. Cortisol deactivates expression of inflammatory genes encoding proinflammatory mediators including cytokines, chemokines, adhesion molecules, inflammatory enzymes, and receptors, whereas it stimulates expression of anti-inflammatory cytokines and chemokines, resulting in decreased inflammation [54].

In the main genomic mechanism, the sequence of GR response element GGAACAnnnTGTTCT is a flawed palindrome that is composed of two 6-base-pair half sites, enabling GR binding as a homodimer. The three nucleotides between the two half sites are necessary for dimerization. Positive GRE refers to GRE that mediates the glucocorticoid-dependent stimulation of targeted genes. While a negative GRE (nGRE) has a specific sequence CTCC(n)0-2GGAGA, it differs from the classical GRE sequence. This sequence is characterized by variable spacer ranging from 0 to 2 and is occupied by 2 GR monomers that do not homodimerize, revealing the complexity of glucocorticoid-mediated gene regulation [48].

The complexity of genomic mechanism extends to the recruitment of co-regulators and chromatin-modifying GC-GR complexes that regulate gene transcription rates. Steroid receptor coactivators (SRC1-3) and histone acetyltransferases CBP/p300, and the nuclear methylase coactivator-associated arginine methyltransferase (CARM1) are cofactors mediating the activation of transcription, while NCoR and SMRT are corepressors that recruit GR bound to nGREs. The majority of GR-binding sites are found outside the promoters of glucocorticoid-responsive genes in intergenic or intragenic regions, showing considerable distance from transcription start sites, indicating that these regulatory elements can accumulate around promoter areas to influence gene transcription *via* three-dimensional chromatin interactions [48].

3.3 Non-genomic effects

Some therapeutic glucocorticoid actions, including bronchodilation and inflammation suppression, happen very quickly to result from transcription, which indicates non-genomic GR effects. This non-specific interaction with cellular membranes and membrane-bound GR functions or specific interaction with cytoplasmic GR causes posttranslational changes, such as phosphorylation. Non-genomic mechanisms have been discovered in epithelial cells in the lung, T-cells, and macrophages [55]. These mechanisms account for many of cortisol's sustained effects; the hormone also exerts rapid non-genomic effects that occur within seconds to minutes rather than hours. These rapid actions run through membrane-bound receptors and signaling molecule that involve secondary messengers, leading to the stimulation of various cellular processes, such as ion transport, neurotransmitter release, and immune cell function without requiring changes in gene expression.

There are signs confirming non-genomic mechanisms, producing quick cellular responses that bypass classical transcriptional mechanisms. These mechanisms ultimately affect the activity of various protein kinases, such as adenylate cyclase-cAMP-PKA, PI3K/AKT, and MAPKs, generating direct and fast cellular responses that match responses from the slower genomic mechanisms [56–58]. The rapid inhibitory effect in *C. punctatus* is mediated by cortisol through adenylate cyclase-cAMP-PKA. This rapid mechanism needs a 15-minute exposure to suppress phagocytosis, while the traditional transcriptional mechanism requires 1–3-hour exposure to inhibit phagocytic activity [56]. The glucocorticoid-dependent production of certain kinase proteins, including c-Src, can trigger kinase cascades, resulting in annexin 1 phosphorylation and inhibition of cytoplasmic phospholipase A_2 activity [48]. Furthermore, GR has been reported to localize at the plasma membrane within specialized lipid rafts called caveolae-1 (Cav-1). In this plasma membrane location, GR can regulate gap junction intercellular communication through c-Src activity and rapid MAPK-dependent phosphorylation. For example, in lung epithelial cells, glucocorticoid therapy causes a quick (within 2 min) Cav-1 and protein kinase B/Akt phosphorylation in a Src-dependent approach [59]. This represents how cortisol can influence cellular communication and signaling networks through mechanisms distinct from the traditional transcriptional pathway.

4. Summary and future directions

4.1 Key point review

Cortisol is considered one of the most important components that the body needs to perform its various functions. It plays a central role in immunity, inflammation, and the regulation of the sleep wake cycle, and coordinates metabolic function. This role is carried out effectively because of cortisol's ability to move and distribute smoothly throughout most parts of the body. This is mostly because of certain carrier proteins, such as CBG and albumin, that help to move it intracellularly. These transport proteins play a critical role in regulating cortisol distribution and maintaining stable hormone levels in the circulation. By binding cortisol and releasing it when required, they enhance its bioavailability to target tissues and protect it from rapid metabolic degradation.

Cortisol is transported and distributed by sophisticated delivery system. The dynamic equilibrium between unbound and bound forms of cortisol guarantees proper hormone bioavailability. The tissue-specific expression of 11β-HSD enzymes creates local cortisol concentrations, enabling precise regulation of glucocorticoid effects independent of cortisol concentration in the circulation, allowing local tissues to modify their cortisol exposure based on their specific demands.

Furthermore, the cortisol-receptor complex moves to the nucleus, where it interacts with GREs in DNA and controls transcription. In this way, cortisol changes the transcription of many genes that are important for different cellular functions. In addition to these classical genomic effects, emerging evidence suggests that cortisol also participates in non-genomic mechanisms, including modulation of intracellular signaling pathways and post-translational modification processes. The integration of rapid non-genomic effects with traditional transcription effects allows cortisol to exert and organize quick stress responses, at the same time keeping long-standing homeostatic tasks. This dual mechanism explains cortisol's capacity to address both acute physiological requests and chronic-adjusted needs. These findings highlight the complex and multifaceted nature of cortisol signaling in cellular physiology.

4.2 Emerging research areas

Advanced knowledge of cortisol's circadian rhythm and equilibrium dynamics is essential for repairing interrupted cortisol rhythms through time-programmed styles according to physiological patterns that are ideal for individual circadian phenotypes. The precise quantification of cortisol in biological samples represents a fundamental requirement for clarifying stress-related physiological mechanisms and improving the accuracy of diagnosis. Classical diagnostic approaches for cortisol measurement have some technical limits, raising the needs to improve modern detection methods. Electrochemical sensing technique has revealed dependable way for point-of-care cortisol analysis, enabling quick diagnostic tool beyond traditional laboratory settings [60].

Preclinical studies on the human microbiome have explained the theory of a brain-gut microbiome axis. This showed a bidirectional interaction between nervous system and gut microbial ecosystems, enabling to identify novel drug targets for brain-gut illnesses [61]. Currently, nanoparticle prodrugs and nanoconjugates are used to deliver glucocorticoids, enabling control of glucocorticoid administration. This nanoparticle-based delivery technique facilitates a precise distribution of glucocorticoids to the targeted tissues and reduces glucocorticoid systemic distribution. The advanced strategy of glucocorticoid prodrugs and conjugates addresses the persistent clinical challenge of augmenting treatment benefits and alleviating the complications associated with glucocorticoid therapy [62].

Author's contributions

B.D.A. contributed to chapter proposal and main concept, and chapter plan and design; B.D.A., T.A.S., and M.H.A. wrote and edited the first draft of the chapter; B.D.A., T.A.S., M.H.A., and A.M.A. revised the first draft of the chapter, and all authors read the final version of the chapter and agreed to submit it.

Funding

This scientific work received no external funding.

Conflict of interest

The authors declare no conflict of interest.

Author details

Bandar D. Alrehaili*, Tahani A. Saeedi, Mohammed H. Alsubhi and Ali M. Alalawi
Department of Pharmacology and Toxicology, College of Pharmacy, Taibah University, Medinah, Saudi Arabia

*Address all correspondence to: brehaili@taibahu.edu.sa

References

[1] MacDougall-Shackleton SA et al. Glucocorticoids and "stress" are not synonymous. Integrative Organismal Biology. 2019;**1**(1):18

[2] Lovallo WR. Cortisol secretion patterns in addiction and addiction risk. International Journal of Psychophysiology. 2006;**59**(3):195-202

[3] Bradbury MJ, Akana SF, Dallman MF. Roles of type I and II corticosteroid receptors in regulation of basal activity in the hypothalamo-pituitary-adrenal axis during the diurnal trough and the peak: Evidence for a nonadditive effect of combined receptor occupation. Endocrinology. 1994;**134**(3):1286-1296

[4] Hamidi O et al. Cortisol testing to diagnose adrenal insufficiency following adrenalectomy for mild autonomous cortisol secretion. The Journal of Clinical Endocrinology & Metabolism. 2025;**111**(3):665-678

[5] George MY et al. The cortisol axis and psychiatric disorders: An updated review. Pharmacological Reports. 2025;**77**(6):1573-1599

[6] O'Byrne NA et al. Sleep and circadian regulation of cortisol: A short review. Current Opinion in Endocrine and Metabolic Research. 2021;**18**:178-186

[7] Liu PY. Rhythms in cortisol mediate sleep and circadian impacts on health. Sleep. 2024;**47**(9):1-3

[8] Poomthavorn P et al. Serum free cortisol index, free cortisol, and total cortisol in critically ill children. Intensive Care Medicine. 2009;**35**(7):1281-1285

[9] Young EA, Abelson J, Lightman SL. Cortisol pulsatility and its role in stress regulation and health. Frontiers in Neuroendocrinology. 2004;**25**(2):69-76

[10] Herman JP et al. Brain mechanisms of HPA axis regulation: Neurocircuitry and feedback in context Richard Kvetnansky lecture. Stress. 2020;**23**(6):617-632

[11] Gjerstad JK, Lightman SL, Spiga F. Role of glucocorticoid negative feedback in the regulation of HPA axis pulsatility. Stress. 2018;**21**(5):403-416

[12] Oster H et al. The functional and clinical significance of the 24-hour rhythm of circulating glucocorticoids. Endocrine Reviews. 2016;**38**(1):3-45

[13] Androulakis IP. Circadian rhythms and the HPA axis: A systems view. WIREs Mechanisms of Disease. 2021;**13**(4):e1518

[14] Patton AP, Hastings MH. The suprachiasmatic nucleus. Current Biology. 2018;**28**(15):R816-R822

[15] Wust S et al. The cortisol awakening response-normal values and confounds. Noise and Health. 2000;**2**(7):79-88

[16] Elder GJ et al. The cortisol awakening response – Applications and implications for sleep medicine. Sleep Medicine Reviews. 2014;**18**(3):215-224

[17] Vgontzas AN et al. Rapid eye movement sleep correlates with the overall activities of the hypothalamic-pituitary-adrenal axis and sympathetic system in healthy humans. The Journal of Clinical Endocrinology & Metabolism. 1997;**82**(10):3278-3280

[18] Bierwolf C et al. Slow wave sleep drives inhibition of pituitary-adrenal secretion in humans. Journal of Neuroendocrinology. 1997;**9**(6):479-484

[19] Mohd Azmi NAS et al. Cortisol on circadian rhythm and its effect on cardiovascular system. International Journal of Environmental Research and Public Health. 2021;**18**(2):676

[20] Andreadi A et al. Modified cortisol circadian rhythm: The hidden toll of night-shift work. International Journal of Molecular Sciences. 2025;**26**(5):2090

[21] Manenschijn L et al. Shift work at young age is associated with elevated long-term cortisol levels and body mass index. The Journal of Clinical Endocrinology & Metabolism. 2011;**96**(11):E1862-E1865

[22] Wilhelm I et al. Is the cortisol awakening rise a response to awakening? Psychoneuroendocrinology. 2007;**32**(4):358-366

[23] Gatti R et al. Cortisol assays and diagnostic laboratory procedures in human biological fluids. Clinical Biochemistry. 2009;**42**(12):1205-1217

[24] Deutschbein T et al. Salivary cortisol as a diagnostic tool for Cushing's syndrome and adrenal insufficiency: Improved screening by an automatic immunoassay. European Journal of Endocrinology. 2012;**166**(4):613-618

[25] Raff H, Raff JL, Findling JW. Late-night salivary cortisol as a screening test for Cushing's syndrome. The Journal of Clinical Endocrinology & Metabolism. 1998;**83**(8):2681-2686

[26] Imani MM et al. Associations between morning salivary and blood cortisol concentrations in individuals with obstructive sleep apnea syndrome: A meta-analysis. Frontiers in Endocrinology. 2021;**11**:568823

[27] Henley D, Lightman S, Carrell R. Cortisol and CBG—Getting cortisol to the right place at the right time. Pharmacology & Therapeutics. 2016;**166**:128-135

[28] Choi MH. Clinical and technical aspects in free cortisol measurement. Endocrinology and Metabolism. 2022;**37**(4):599-607

[29] Perogamvros I et al. Corticosteroid-binding globulin regulates cortisol pharmacokinetics. Clinical Endocrinology. 2011;**74**(1):30-36

[30] Pardridge WM, Mietus LJ. Transport of steroid hormones through the rat blood-brain barrier: Primary role of albumin-bound hormone. The Journal of Clinical Investigation. 1979;**64**(1):145-154

[31] Mason BL et al. Central nervous system (CNS) delivery of glucocorticoids is fine-tuned by saturable transporters at the blood-CNS barriers and nonbarrier regions. Endocrinology. 2010;**151**(11):5294-5305

[32] Lewis JG et al. Plasma free cortisol fraction reflects levels of functioning corticosteroid-binding globulin. Clinica Chimica Acta. 2005;**359**(1):189-194

[33] Le Rouzic P, Rousseau K. Binding for life: Corticosteroid binding globulin from vertebrate physiology to human diseases. Frontiers in Endocrinology. 2025;**16**:1647096

[34] Lee JH et al. Corticosteroid-binding globulin (CBG): Spatiotemporal distribution of cortisol in sepsis. Trends in Endocrinology & Metabolism. 2023;**34**(3):181-190

[35] Ramsay SD et al. Harnessing native corticosteroid-binding globulin to treat life-threatening septic shock. Endocrinology. 2026;**167**(2):1-18

[36] Cizza G, Rother KI. Cortisol Binding Globulin: More than Just a Carrier? The Journal of Clinical Endocrinology & Metabolism. 2012;**97**(1):77-80

[37] Musayeva F, Abdullayeva N. The hormone cortisol and its biological role in metabolic disorders. Nature & Science. 2025;**7**(6):9-13

[38] Pardridge WM. Transport of protein-bound hormones into tissues in vivo. Endocrine Reviews. 1981;**2**(1):103-123

[39] Bikle DD. The free hormone hypothesis: When, why, and how to measure the free hormone levels to assess vitamin D, thyroid, sex hormone, and cortisol status. Journal of Bone and Mineral Research Plus. 2021;**5**(1):e10418

[40] Perogamvros I, Ray DW, Trainer PJ. Regulation of cortisol bioavailability—Effects on hormone measurement and action. Nature Reviews Endocrinology. 2012;**8**(12):717-727

[41] Nader N et al. Mitotane has an estrogenic effect on sex hormone-binding globulin and corticosteroid-binding globulin in humans. The Journal of Clinical Endocrinology & Metabolism. 2006;**91**(6):2165-2170

[42] Qureshi AC et al. The influence of the route of oestrogen administration on serum levels of cortisol-binding globulin and total cortisol. Clinical Endocrinology. 2007;**66**(5):632-635

[43] Dichtel LE et al. Plasma free cortisol in states of normal and altered binding globulins: Implications for adrenal insufficiency diagnosis. The Journal of Clinical Endocrinology & Metabolism. 2019;**104**(10):4827-4836

[44] Dorin RI, Qualls CR. Distribution of cortisol in human plasma in vitro: Equilibrium solutions for free cortisol using equations of mass conservation and mass action [Internet]. In: Cortisol-between Physiology and Pathology. London, UK: IntechOpen; 2024. DOI: 10.5772/intechopen.1003598

[45] Stomby A et al. Tissue-specific dysregulation of cortisol regeneration by 11βHSD1 in obesity: Has it promised too much? Diabetologia. 2014;**57**(6):1100-1110

[46] Thau L, Gandhi J, Sharma S. Physiology, cortisol. In: StatPearls [Internet]. Treasure Island (FL): StatPearls Publishing; 2023. Available from: https://www.ncbi.nlm.nih.gov/sites/books/NBK538239/

[47] Kumar R, Thompson EB. Gene regulation by the glucocorticoid receptor: Structure: Function relationship. The Journal of Steroid Biochemistry and Molecular Biology. 2005;**94**(5):383-394

[48] Oakley RH, Cidlowski JA. The biology of the glucocorticoid receptor: New signaling mechanisms in health and disease. Journal of Allergy and Clinical Immunology. 2013;**132**(5):1033-1044

[49] Mangelsdorf DJ et al. The nuclear receptor superfamily: The second decade. Cell. 1995;**83**(6):835-839

[50] Evans RM. The steroid and thyroid hormone receptor superfamily. Science. 1988;**240**(4854):889-895

[51] Nettles KW, Greene GL. Ligand control of coregulator recruitment to nuclear receptors. Annual Review of Physiology. 2005;**67**(1):309-333

[52] Franchimont D. Overview of the actions of glucocorticoids on the immune response: A good model to characterize new pathways of immunosuppression for new treatment strategies. Annals of the New York Academy of Sciences. 2004;**1024**(1):124-137

[53] Rhen T, Cidlowski JA. Antiinflammatory action of glucocorticoids—New mechanisms for old drugs. New England Journal of Medicine. 2005;**353**(16):1711-1723

[54] Chinenov Y et al. Role of transcriptional coregulator GRIP1 in the anti-inflammatory actions of glucocorticoids. Proceedings of the National Academy of Sciences. 2012;**109**(29):11776-11781

[55] Escoter-Torres L et al. Fighting the fire: Mechanisms of inflammatory gene regulation by the glucocorticoid receptor. Frontiers in Immunology. 2019;**10**:1859

[56] Roy B, Rai U. Genomic and non-genomic effect of cortisol on phagocytosis in freshwater teleost Channa punctatus: An in vitro study. Steroids. 2009;**74**(4-5, 455):449

[57] Miller AL et al. p38 mitogen-activated protein kinase (MAPK) is a key mediator in glucocorticoid-induced apoptosis of lymphoid cells: Correlation between p38 MAPK activation and site-specific phosphorylation of the human glucocorticoid receptor at serine 211. Molecular Endocrinology. 2005;**19**(6):1569-1583

[58] Newby EA et al. Adrenocorticotropic hormone and PI3K/Akt inhibition reduce eNOS phosphorylation and increase cortisol biosynthesis in long-term hypoxic ovine fetal adrenal cortical cells. Reproductive Sciences. 2015;**22**(8):932-941

[59] Panettieri RA et al. Non-genomic effects of glucocorticoids: An updated view. Trends in Pharmacological Sciences. 2019;**40**(1):38-49

[60] Karuppaiah G et al. Electrochemical sensors for cortisol detection: Principles, designs, fabrication, and characterisation. Biosensors and Bioelectronics. 2023;**239**:115600

[61] Osadchiy V, Martin CR, Mayer EA. The gut–brain axis and the microbiome: Mechanisms and clinical implications. Clinical Gastroenterology and Hepatology. 2019;**17**(2):322-332

[62] Tessier B et al. Emerging nanoparticle platforms to improve the administration of glucocorticoids. Journal of Controlled Release. 2023;**358**:273-292

Chapter 3

Cortisol: Metabolism

Abdulrahman G. Alharbi and Bandar D. Alrehaili

Abstract

Cortisol is a vital glucocorticoid hormone synthesized by the adrenal cortex. It plays important functions in maintaining metabolic homeostasis and coordinating physiological responses to stress. This chapter provides a comprehensive review of cortisol metabolism, encompassing its synthesis through the hypothalamic-pituitary-adrenal (HPA) axis, steroidogenic pathways, and circadian regulation. The complex transport mechanisms involving corticosteroid-binding globulin and albumin ensure appropriate hormone distribution, while the free hormone hypothesis governs tissue accessibility and biological activity. Cortisol exerts its effects through precise cellular mechanisms involving glucocorticoid receptors, operating via both genomic and non-genomic pathways to regulate gene expression and cellular signaling. The hormone's metabolic effects span glucose homeostasis through gluconeogenesis and glycogen regulation, protein catabolism for amino acid mobilization, and lipolysis with characteristic fat redistribution patterns. These actions are coordinated through complex interactions with insulin and other hormonal systems. Cortisol clearance occurs primarily through hepatic metabolism and 11β-hydroxysteroid dehydrogenase enzyme systems, which provide tissue-specific modulation of glucocorticoid activity. Clinical implications are profound, with hypercortisolism leading to metabolic syndrome and cardiovascular complications, while hypocortisolism results in life-threatening metabolic instability. Understanding cortisol metabolism is essential for developing targeted therapeutic interventions and optimizing treatment strategies for endocrine disorders while minimizing adverse effects.

Keywords: adrenal cortex, adrenocorticotropic hormone, cortisol, cortisol metabolism, hypothalamic-pituitary-adrenal axis, 11β-hydroxysteroid dehydrogenase

1. Introduction

1.1 An overview of cortisol as a glucocorticoid hormone

Cortisol is a natural and principal steroidal hormone of the glucocorticoid class in human and most mammals. It is synthesized from cholesterol and released by the adrenal gland into the bloodstream. Cortisol acts on glucocorticoid receptors which cause different physiological effects. Its synthesis is controlled by the hypothalamic-pituitary-adrenal (HPA) axis [1, 2], the body's main neuro-endocrine system regulating stress responses (detailed in Section 2.1). Glucocorticoids appear to enhance

IntechOpen

activity in various brain regions, such as the amygdala [3, 4], suggesting site-specific effects of glucocorticoid stimulation that influence the behavioral and cognitive functions associated with these areas.

Cortisol is commonly termed as "stress hormone" due to its physiological roles which results in stress responses leading to essential regulatory functions across multiple organ systems [5]. Cortisol mediates adaptive responses to diverse stimuli that disturb homeostasis, from psychological stressors to physical challenges. It also demonstrates anti-inflammatory effects across multiple tissues and concurrently regulates metabolism in muscle, adipose tissue, liver, and bone [6]. Cortisol modulates mood, behavior, and sleep-wake cycles within the central nervous system [7]. Cortisol's regulatory capacity allows it to induce essential behavioral, cognitive, and physiological adaptations to regulate stressors and challenges, establishing it as a key coordinator of the body's stress response rather than simply a stress indicator [1]. Cortisol can also influence vascular tone through its effects on the autonomic nervous and cardiovascular systems [7], leading to enhance the vasoconstrictor action of adrenergic stimuli on small blood vessels. Thus, cortisol is considered as a key coordinator of the body's stress response rather than simply a stress indicator [1].

Secretion of cortisol follows an evolutionarily conserved circadian rhythm [8]. This temporal organization is featured by peak cortisol levels in the early morning hours, followed by a gradual reduction throughout the day, reaching its lowest concentrations during the evening and early night-time hours, a pattern that synchronizes metabolic and physiological processes with the sleep-wake cycle. This circadian rhythm ensures cortisol level is maintained under normal conditions to avoid unwanted stress responses.

Cortisol levels are chronically increased in conditions like Cushing's disease or when administration of exogenous glucocorticoids [9]. The high levels of cortisol can generally be found in chronic stress settings that leads to disruption of organ functions which include metabolic dysfunction, cardiovascular problems, visceral obesity, hepatic steatosis, bone demineralization, immunosuppression, and neuropsychiatric diseases such as mood disorders and sleep disturbances [5].

The adverse outcomes highlight the significance of the HPA axis's complex control mechanisms, which utilize negative feedback loops to regulate cortisol levels effectively. The regulatory system ensures that increased glucocorticoid levels inhibit the release of upstream corticotropin-releasing hormone (CRH) and adrenocorticotropic hormone (ACTH), resulting in a pulsatile secretion pattern that spikes in the early morning and supports a healthy circadian rhythm.

1.2 Importance of cortisol in human physiology

Cortisol's essential physiological functions include vital regulatory mechanisms that preserve homeostatic balance. The morning surge of the hormone increases vascular tone and alertness, mobilizes energy reserves, and prepares the immune system for optimal function [1]. This coordinated activation prepares the body for daily challenges. During stress, heightened glucocorticoid secretion from the adrenal glands creates sustained cortisol elevations that trigger more intense physiological responses. For example, in a 'fight or flight' scenario, cortisol increases vascular tone and alertness, raising plasma glucose to provide energy for physical exertion, and prepares the immune system for potential harm [6, 10]. The anticipatory effects enhance the likelihood of successfully managing the stressor, thereby promoting a rapid restoration of homeostasis.

Cortisol serves as a potent immunosuppressive hormone which inhibits the immune system by reducing the circulation of lymphocytes [11]. This compromises the body's ability to fight infections. In addition, cortisol is a potent anti-inflammatory agent which inhibits the production of proinflammatory signaling molecules such as cytokines and chemokines in injured tissue. These mediators trigger the immune cells by direct cellular effects in damaged tissues. Herein, cortisol directly impacts immune cells by hindering their ability to infiltrate tissue as well as in certain cell types, it induces apoptosis. Cortisol promotes the activation of scavenger immune cells resulting in removing cellular debris, improving healing processes, and preventing long-term damage, such as fibrosis [11]. Cortisol modulates cellular metabolism, adhesion, migration, and survival in a manner specific to both the cell type and its surroundings.

The balance of cortisol's functions across various physiological pathways underscores its importance in human physiology. The function extends beyond a simple stress response; it encompasses a complex network of regulatory mechanisms that maintain homeostasis across multiple bodily systems. Given cortisol's central role in human physiology, this chapter provides a comprehensive review of its metabolism from synthesis to clearance, with emphasis on clinical implications.

1.3 Chapter scope and objectives

The objective of this chapter is to offer readers an in-depth understanding of cortisol metabolism, encompassing molecular mechanisms and clinical applications. The scope includes each aspect of cortisol biology, starting with its synthesis and regulation via the HPA axis, and advancing through cellular mechanisms, metabolic effects, and clearance pathways.

In this chapter, the HPA axis controls mechanisms, and the steroidogenic pathway will be elucidated to highlight how cortisol production is precisely controlled under physiological conditions. The chapter includes a comprehensively review of cortisol's effect on glucose metabolism, protein catabolism, lipolysis, and interactions with other hormonal systems that collectively regulate metabolic homeostasis. The pathophysiology of cortisol dysregulation, and therapeutic interventions will be mentioned in several sections of this chapter.

Upon completing this chapter, readers will have a thorough understanding of cortisol metabolism, allowing them to better understand its physiological significance, identify pathological changes, and comprehend the reasoning beyond therapeutic strategies aimed at glucocorticoid pathways.

2. Cortisol synthesis

2.1 Hypothalamic-pituitary-adrenal (HPA) axis regulation

The production and release of cortisol are regulated by the HPA axis. Upon experiencing a stress, the hypothalamus secretes CRH, which then transits to the anterior pituitary gland via the hypophyseal portal system. The pituitary gland releases ACTH into the bloodstream, stimulating the middle zona fasciculata of adrenal cortex to produce and release cortisol [2].

The HPA axis comprises three basic structures that regulate the stress response: the paraventricular nucleus (PVN) of the hypothalamus [12], the anterior pituitary gland, and the adrenal cortex [13]. These structures work together to regulate adrenal hormones, which aid in maintaining or restoring homeostasis. The activation of the HPA axis begins when hypophysiotropic neurons in the PVN of the hypothalamus are stimulated to produce and release CRH and arginine vasopressin (AVP). CRH and AVP are released into the median eminence and subsequently transported to the anterior pituitary gland via the hypophyseal portal vessels. Upon reaching the anterior pituitary gland, CRH interacts with corticotropin receptor factor type 1 receptors (CRFR1), located on the corticotropic cells. This interaction results in the synthesis of ACTH from pre-pro-opiomelanocortin (pre-POMC) and triggers the secretion of ACTH into the systemic circulation [13].

Under normal conditions, the anterior pituitary gland secretes ACTH in regular pulses of varying amplitude daily. ACTH levels exhibit an endogenous circadian rhythm similar to cortisol, peaking in the morning and decreasing throughout the day. The relationship between ACTH and the production of cortisol is regulated by negative feedback to the anterior pituitary to suppress additional ACTH release, thereby preventing sustained elevations in cortisol levels [14]. ACTH is secreted in a pulsatile manner, influencing cortisol secretion through the regulation of gene transcription for key enzymes involved in steroidogenesis. These include steroidogenic acute regulatory protein (STAR), cytochrome P450 side-chain cleavage (P450scc), as well as the MC2R and its accessory protein (MRAP) [14, 15].

2.2 Steroidogenic pathway

The steroidogenic pathway for cortisol synthesis represents a complicated series of enzymatic reactions. It begins with cholesterol that actively transported into adrenal gland via LDL receptors [16]. Inside the adrenal cell, the critical rate-limiting step involves the movement of cholesterol from the exterior to the interior of the mitochondrial membrane, facilitated by the steroidogenic acute regulatory protein (STAR) [17]. This protein-mediated transport is thought to be as the main regulatory point for acute steroidogenesis and found to demonstrate a strong response to ACTH stimulation [17]. The vital significance of this step is demonstrated by the fact that congenital lipoid adrenal hyperplasia is linked to STAR protein dysfunction [16].

Following successful cholesterol transport, the steroidogenic cascade proceeds through a series of sequential enzymatic conversions. The initial enzymatic conversion is mediated by CYP11A1, which breaks the cholesterol side chain to produce pregnenolone. This irreversible reaction constitutes the initial committed step in steroidogenesis, necessitating molecular oxygen and nicotinamide adenine dinucleotide phosphate (NADPH) as substrates [18].

The pathway then continues as pregnenolone is subsequently subjected to 17α-hydroxylation by CYP17A1, a bifunctional enzyme that exhibits both hydroxylase and lyase activities. Hydroxylase activity is crucial for cortisol synthesis, whereas lyase activity is vital for androgen production [18]. This dual functionality allows the pathway to branch toward different steroid hormones depending on tissue-specific needs.

3β-Hydroxysteroid dehydrogenase (3β-HSD) converts 17α-hydroxypregnenolone to 17α-hydroxyprogesterone through oxidation and isomerization reactions. Deficiency in this enzyme causes congenital adrenal hyperplasia with variable salt-wasting and virilization.

Progressing toward cortisol completion, the enzyme CYP21A2 (21-hydroxylase), which is essential to produce both glucocorticoids and mineralocorticoids, mediates the subsequent conversion to 11-deoxycortisol. CYP21A2 deficiency represents the predominant etiology of congenital adrenal hyperplasia, underscoring its clinical importance [19]. Finally, the ultimate step in cortisol biosynthesis occurs when CYP11B1 (11β-hydroxylase) catalyzes the final hydroxylation to produce cortisol (**Figure 1**). This enzyme is primarily expressed in the zona fasciculata and dependent on ACTH stimulation [20].

ACTH regulation of steroidogenesis (see Section 2.1) occurs through melanocortin-2 receptor binding on adrenocortical cells, activating adenylyl cyclase and elevating intracellular cAMP levels to stimulate protein kinase A. This cascade enhances

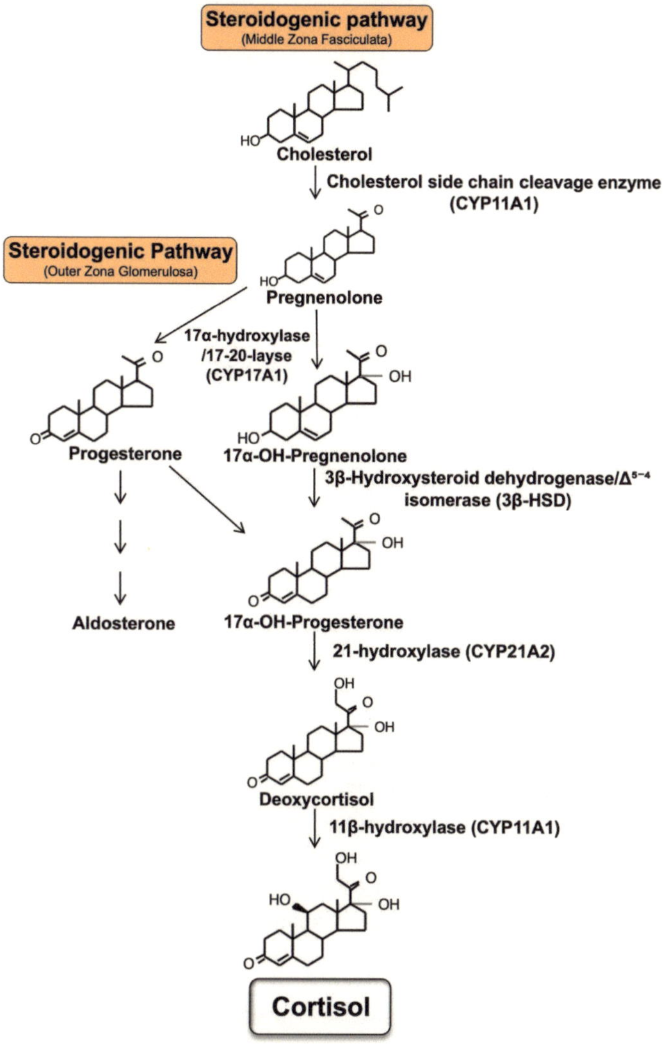

Figure 1.
Synthesis of cortisol in adrenal cortex. The steroidogenic pathway is started with the action of CYP11A1 which cleave side chain of cholesterol to create pregnenolone. Through an additional enzymatic reaction, 17α-hydroxypregnenolone and progesterone are synthesized. Subsequently, these two products are converted into 17α-hydroxyprogesterone by oxidation and hydroxylation reactions, respectively. Then, dexoycortisol is synthesized by 21-hydroxylase (CYP21A2). Cortisol is produced by action of 11β-hydroxylase (CYP11B1) in the final step.

both acute steroidogenesis (STAR activation) and chronic production (transcriptional upregulation of steroidogenic enzymes) [14, 15, 20].

Comprehending this intricate pathway and its regulation is crucial for the diagnosis and treatment of adrenal disorders, specifically congenital adrenal hyperplasia and Cushing's syndrome, which exemplify the extremes of cortisol metabolism dysfunction.

3. Metabolic effects

The cellular mechanisms of cortisol lead to coordinated metabolic changes that increase resistance to physiological or pathological stresses through sustain release of energy. Cortisol regulates a metabolic response across various target tissues, emphasizing glucose availability and mobilizing protein and lipid reserves to supply energy during elevated physiological necessities.

3.1 Glucose metabolism

The regulation of glucose homeostasis represents one of the cortisol's most critical metabolic functions, with the hormone exerting comprehensive effects across multiple target tissues to raise blood glucose levels during stress and fasting states [1]. Cortisol's predominantly catabolic effects favor the liberation of energy stores, which proves its role to stabilize trauma, fright, and illness, while simultaneously coordinating metabolic responses across hepatic, muscular, adipose, and pancreatic tissues to ensure adequate glucose availability for vital organ function to resist stress.

3.1.1 Effects of cortisol on hepatic gluconeogenesis and glycogenesis

In the liver, cortisol has gluconeogenic and glycogenic effects that act as the primary mechanisms for preserving systemic glucose availability. It exerts its gluconeogenic effects primarily by stimulating the expression of rate-limiting enzymes, particularly phosphoenolpyruvate carboxykinase (PEPCK) and glucose-6-phosphatase. PEPCK catalyzes the conversion of oxaloacetate to phosphoenolpyruvate, the rate-limiting step in gluconeogenesis, while glucose-6-phosphatase enables the final glucose release from hepatocytes [21]. Cortisol also upregulates fructose-1,6-bisphosphatase and pyruvate carboxylase, creating a coordinated enzymatic response that maximizes hepatic glucose production. These enzymatic regulations occur through cortisol-induced glucocorticoid receptor binding to glucocorticoid response elements within the promoter regions of genes encoding these enzymes, representing the fundamental mechanism of cortisol's transcriptional control over glucose production [21]. Cortisol can also stimulate hepatic glycogen formation through increased hepatic glycogen synthase activity. This results in creating glucose reserves that can be rapidly mobilized during subsequent metabolic demands. Thus, roles of cortisol in these two major metabolic pathways maintain glucose homeostasis during periods of stress or fasting.

The metabolic significance of cortisol-mediated gluconeogenesis extends beyond simple glucose production, as it coordinates with other catabolic processes including lipolysis and protein degradation to ensure adequate substrate availability [22]. This integrated response reveals cortisol's task in energy redistribution during stress, where glucose becomes the ideal fuel for critical organs, particularly the brain and immune system. However, chronic activation of this pathway contributes significantly to the hyperglycemic manifestations observed in hypercortisolemic states such as Cushing's syndrome.

3.1.2 Effects of cortisol on skeletal muscle and glycogen storage

Cortisol's effects on skeletal muscle reveal its essential function in redirecting metabolic substrates from peripheral tissues to support central glucose production. Cortisol impairs insulin-stimulated glycogen synthesis by decreasing muscle glycogen synthase activity and fostering insulin resistance through gene regulation of glucocorticoid receptor that involve in the insulin-signaling cascade. This results in post-receptor defects with reduced downstream phosphoinositide-3-kinase and AKT activities [21]. Furthermore, cortisol stimulates glycogenolysis in muscle through epinephrine-induced activation of glycogen phosphorylase and promotes the generation of gluconeogenic precursors by facilitating lipolysis of triglyceride stores and protein degradation in muscle tissue [23].

The effects of cortisol on glycogen metabolism exhibit complex tissue-specific actions that reflect the hormone's dual role in energy mobilization and storage. Cortisol's hepatic effects contrast markedly with cortisol's actions in skeletal muscle. This illustrates how tissue-specific nature of cortisol's glycogen effects reflects the differential expression and activity of 11β-HSD enzymes to modulate local cortisol concentrations and receptor activation. In pathological conditions characterized by insulin resistance, cortisol's capacity to promote hepatic glycogenesis becomes impaired which results in glucose homeostasis disruption and development of type 2 diabetes mellitus.

3.1.3 Effects of cortisol on adipose tissue and pancreatic function

Cortisol regulates several mechanisms in adipocytes leading to complex metabolic changes. It downregulates glucose transporter type 4 (GLUT4) expression which reduces insulin-stimulated glucose uptake by 40–60%. Simultaneously, cortisol prevents key glycolytic enzymes including hexokinase and phosphofructokinase while stimulating gluconeogenic enzyme expression, effectively converting adipose tissue from a glucose-consuming to glucose-producing organ during stress conditions. It prevents glucose uptake and oxidation while promoting lipolysis to provide glycerol as a precursor for hepatic gluconeogenesis [21]. These mechanisms contributing to decreased glucose utilization by cortisol in adipocytes involve modulation of GLUT4 function and disruption of insulin signaling cascades [21]. Additionally, cortisol participates in the differentiation and expansion of adipocyte precursors that are fundamental in a process that may further intensify insulin resistance and adipocyte dysfunction [24].

Cortisol acts as a counter-regulatory hormone to insulin and potentially creates conditions that promote insulin resistance. It impairs glucose-stimulated insulin secretion by promoting the degradation of glucose transporter (GLUT4) in pancreatic β-cells and reducing glucokinase expression levels [21]. Moreover, cortisol increases glucose-6-phosphatase activity leading to reduce the entry of glucose-6-phosphate into the glycolytic cycle and simultaneously induce glucagon secretion in pancreatic α-cells [21]. During high levels of cortisol and effect of negative feedback mechanism, glycogenesis pathway is inhibited, and glucose storage is depleted by the liver as glycogen becomes reduced, contributing to hyperglycemic effects that observed in hypercortisolemic states.

3.2 Protein catabolism and amino acid mobilization

Effects of cortisol on protein catabolism represent a fundamental component of the stress response. These cortisol's catabolic effects primarily disturb peripheral tissues such as skeletal muscle, lymphoid, and connective tissues while generally preserving hepatic and cardiac protein contents. In skeletal muscle, cortisol stimulates proteolysis through activation of the ubiquitin-proteasome pathway, especially E3 ligases including atrogin-1 (MuRF1) [25]. This catabolic process releases branched-chain amino acids (e.g., leucine, isoleucine, and valine) and alanine, which serve as gluconeogenic substrates in hepatic glucose production.

The mobilization of amino acids by cortisol involves sophisticated transport and metabolic conversion mechanisms that ensure efficient substrate delivery to hepatic gluconeogenic pathways. Cortisol enhances amino acid uptake by hepatic tissue through upregulation of specific amino acid transporters, facilitating the conversion of amino acids to glucose via transamination and deamination reactions. The alanine-glucose cycle represents a particularly important component of this system, whereby muscle-derived alanine serves as the primary gluconeogenic substrate in hepatic tissue, effectively transferring nitrogen from peripheral tissues to the liver for urea synthesis and disposal [26].

The clinical significance of cortisol-mediated protein catabolism becomes evident in conditions of chronic cortisol excess, where prolonged exposure leads to progressive muscle wasting, skin thinning, and compromised wound healing. These effects reflect cortisol's preferential targeting of structural proteins in peripheral tissues to maintain glucose availability for vital organ function. This highlights the importance of cortisol in regulating protein and glucose homeostasis.

3.3 Lipolysis and fat redistribution

Cortisol's lipolytic effects show outstanding tissue specificity that promote triglyceride breakdown through activation of hormone-sensitive lipase and adipose triglyceride lipase. However, cortisol can also stimulate lipogenesis which accumulates fat in specific anatomical regions such as face and shoulders [1, 22]. During stress, elevated free fatty acid concentrations due to the cortisol's action on lipolysis serves as alternative fuel sources [24]. These elevated fatty acid levels also contribute to insulin resistance through the Randle cycle mechanism; whereby the stimulation of fatty acid oxidation inhibits glucose utilization in peripheral tissues [27]. The apparent paradox of cortisol simultaneously promoting lipolysis and fat accumulation reflects the complex interaction between cortisol effects and local metabolic conditions. In chronic stress and unrestricted energy intake without corresponding energy expenditure, fatty acid esterification predominates over lipolysis combined with cortisol-stimulated pre-adipocyte differentiation to promote net fat accumulation in specific areas of the body.

Cortisol promotes characteristic patterns of fat redistribution that reflect tissue-specific differences in glucocorticoid receptor density and 11β-hydroxysteroid dehydrogenase type 1 expression [20]. It preferentially promotes visceral abdominal fat accumulation due to the high concentration of glucocorticoid receptors in this anatomical region, while simultaneously promoting the development of dorsocervical fat pads and characteristic facial fat deposition which can be seen in patients with adrenal incidentaloma [28]. This redistribution pattern contrasts with the relative depletion of subcutaneous fat in peripheral regions, particularly the extremities where enhanced lipolysis predominates.

The clinical significance of cortisol-mediated fat redistribution encompasses vital pathophysiological implications beyond physical appearance, as visceral adipose tissue accumulation contributes significantly to metabolic dysfunction through altered adipokine secretion patterns. Cortisol upregulates LIM domain only 3 (LMO3) which is known to influence the expression of 11β-HSD1. Following upregulation of LMO3, adipocyte differentiation is modulated by Peroxisome proliferator-activated receptor gamma (PPARγ) [29]. Cortisol also increases hepatic de novo lipogenesis rates that potentially decrease the available cytosolic triacylglycerol pool. This resulting in elevation of the exported triglycerides into adipose tissues leading to hepatic steatosis.

3.4 Hormonal interactions and metabolic integration

Metabolism of cortisol involves complex interactions with multiple hormonal systems that collectively determine the net metabolic outcomes in target tissues. The cortisol's counter-regulatory relationship with insulin represents one of the most clinically significant of these interactions. Cortisol opposes insulin's anabolic actions on glucose, protein, and lipid metabolisms through multiple mechanisms [22]. These include impairment of insulin signaling pathway through receptor downregulation and post-receptor defects leading to compensatory hyperinsulinemia as β-cells attempt to overcome peripheral insulin resistance.

The interaction between cortisol and growth hormone demonstrates additional complexity in metabolic regulation. Cortisol antagonizes the anabolic effects of growth hormone on protein synthesis and linear growth while simultaneously suppressing insulin-like growth factor-1 production and action [30]. Similarly, cortisol modulates thyroid hormone effects on metabolic rate and thermogenesis. Cortisol also affects peripheral conversion of thyroxine to triiodothyronine and opposes stimulation of protein synthesis via thyroid hormone. These multihormonal interactions highlight the integrated nature of metabolic regulation and explain why disruption of cortisol homeostasis can have widespread metabolic consequences that extend far beyond the direct effects of glucocorticoid receptor activation.

4. Cortisol clearance and inactivation

To prevent excessive accumulation and maintain hormonal equilibrium, cortisol must be efficiently eliminated from the circulation after it has performed its metabolic and physiological effects. The elimination process involves several pathways and enzymatic systems that collaboratively convert cortisol into inactive metabolites for excretion, while also facilitating local modulation of glucocorticoid activity.

4.1 Hepatic cortisol metabolism

The liver serves as the primary site for cortisol biotransformation. It also plays a crucial role in cortisol clearance through the action of various enzymes that metabolize cortisol. Hepatic metabolism of cortisol involves a complex series of reduction, oxidation, and conjugation reactions that transform cortisol into more water-soluble metabolites suitable for excretion [31].

Hepatic cortisol metabolism encompasses multiple enzymatic pathways. A-ring reductases (5α-reductase and 5β-reductase) reduce the C4-C5 double bond, producing 5α-tetrahydrocortisol (5α-THF) and 5β-tetrahydrocortisol (5β-THF), respectively. These represent 70–80% of cortisol metabolites. Additional pathways include 20α- and 20β-hydroxysteroid dehydrogenases producing α- and β-cortols (**Figure 2**) [32]. These reduction reactions represent the rate-limiting steps in cortisol inactivation and demonstrate significant inter-individual variability that may contribute to differential susceptibility to glucocorticoid-related metabolic disorders. This variability explains why some individuals are developing cortisol-related complications even with similar hormone exposures.

4.2 11β-HSD enzymes and cortisol-cortisone interconversion

Beyond the hepatic clearance mechanisms, the interconversion between active cortisol and inactive cortisone is regulated by 11β-hydroxysteroid dehydrogenase (11β-HSD) enzymes, which represent a critical pre-receptor mechanism for modulating local cortisol activity [33]. There are two isoforms of this enzyme with distinct

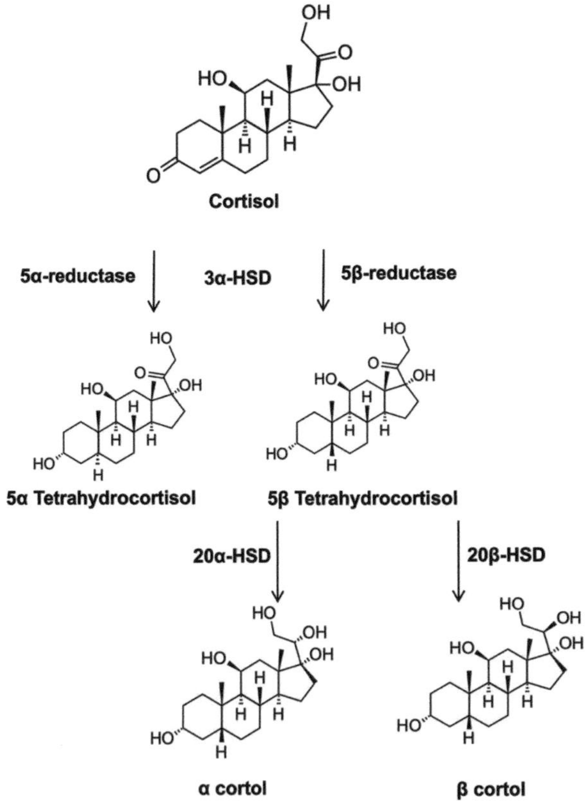

Figure 2.
Degradation of cortisol's metabolites. This diagram shows metabolites degradation of cortisol. The C4-C5 double bonds are reduced via 5α- and 5β- reductase enzymes to produce 5α- and 5β- tetrahydrocortisol, respectively. 5β-tetrahydrocortisol is processed by additional HSD enzymes to create additional metabolites, α- and β cortols.

functions and tissue distribution patterns that collectively determine tissue-specific cortisol exposure. 11β-HSD1 acts as a reductase in vivo, converting cortisone to cortisol using NADPH, thereby increasing local cortisol activity in target tissues such as liver, adipose tissue, bone, and central nervous system (CNS). Co-localization with hexose-6-phosphate dehydrogenase provides necessary NADPH cofactor [1, 22].

Conversely, 11β-HSD2 exclusively dehydrogenates cortisol to cortisone using nicotinamide adenine dinucleotide+ (NAD+), predominantly in mineralocorticoid target tissues (kidney, colon, salivary glands, and placenta) to protect mineralocorticoid receptors from cortisol activation [1]. This tissue-specific expression enables local glucocorticoid activity modulation independent of systemic concentrations.

4.3 Renal cortisol excretion

The kidneys play a major role in the excretion of cortisol metabolites. Renal cortisol elimination represents a minor component of total cortisol clearance under normal physiological conditions. After hepatic metabolism, the water-soluble cortisol metabolites are filtered at the glomerulus and excreted in urine with minimal reabsorption [34]. The measurement of urinary free cortisol and its metabolites serves as a valuable clinical tool for assessing cortisol production and metabolism. This provides insights into both central axis activity and peripheral metabolic capacity.

Previous studies reveal that around 80 to 90% of filtered cortisol is reabsorbed by the renal tubules. This indicates that the kidney serves as a conservation mechanism rather than the primary clearance pathway for cortisol under physiological conditions. This conservation mechanism ensures that physiological cortisol levels are maintained efficiently. For example, urinary cortisol excretion is increased to correlates with normal plasma cortisol concentrations during cortisol excess conditions. This relationship makes urinary cortisol measurements particularly useful for detecting and monitoring hypercortisolemic states [34].

4.4 Cortisol metabolites and their clinical significance

Cortisol metabolites can act as biomarkers for specific enzymatic pathways which they provide insights into cortisol metabolism disorders. The major urinary metabolites of cortisol including 5α-tetrahydrocortisol (5α-THF), 5β-tetrahydrocortisol (5β-THF), 5β-tetrahydrocortisone (5β-THE), cortols, and cortolones, each reflecting different aspects of cortisol biotransformation [32]. High excretion of 5β-THF indicates increased 5β-reductase activity and enhanced cortisol clearance through this pathway (**Figure 2**). The ratio of 5β-THF to cortisol serves as a biomarker of metabolic dysfunction in conditions such as polycystic ovary syndrome. Meanwhile, high levels of 5α-THF reflects peripheral cortisol metabolism. However, this pathway is less quantitatively significant than 5β-reduction for cortisol elimination. This provides important information about steroid metabolism in peripheral tissues and may be altered in insulin resistance states [32].

The pattern of cortisol metabolite excretion provides diagnostic information about enzyme deficiencies, drug interactions, and metabolic disorders. Altered ratios of cortisol metabolites can indicate specific enzymatic abnormalities and help explain discordances between clinical symptoms and circulating cortisol levels. Moreover, these metabolites work as end products for assessing the efficacy of therapeutic interventions that are targeting cortisol metabolism. Thus, excreted metabolites of cortisol are valuable tools for both diagnosis and treatment monitoring in clinical practice.

5. Cortisol dysregulation and clinical implications

The regulatory mechanisms of cortisol metabolism are complicated and can be easily disrupted. This resulting in notable clinical manifestations that highlight cortisol's essential role in human health. Dysregulations offer significant understandings into normal cortisol physiology and underline the challenges and opportunities for therapeutic intervention.

5.1 Clinical assessment and diagnosis

Metabolic cortisol disorders require systematic diagnostic strategies that combine biochemical assessments with clinical manifestations. For example, Late-night salivary cortisol measurement has become the most sensitive screening method for hypercortisolism. Secerning at late night shows a sensitivity greater than 92% and a specificity exceeding 95% in the detection of Cushing's syndrome [21]. This method is more effective than random cortisol measurements as it identifies the disruption of the normal circadian rhythm which is a key indicator of pathological cortisol excess.

Renal free cortisol excretion indicates total cortisol production over a 24-hour period; however, results should be analyzed considering variables influencing cortisol clearance, such as age, body mass, and liver function. The cortisol metabolite profile offers supplementary diagnostic insights, as altered 5α-reductase/5β-reductase ratios suggest specific enzymatic abnormalities that could elucidate discrepancies between symptoms and cortisol levels [35]. The diagnosis of hypocortisolism is based on insufficient cortisol responses to physiological stress that are commonly evaluated via cosyntropin stimulation testing. Peak cortisol responses below 18–20 μg/dL suggest adrenal insufficiency. However, thresholds may need to be modified according to assay techniques and clinical circumstances.

5.2 Hypercortisolism and metabolic syndrome

Cushing's syndrome represents the clinical consequences of chronic hypercortisolism, presenting with characteristic metabolic, cardiovascular, and physical manifestations. Patients develop central obesity with specific fat redistribution patterns. About 40–50% of patients can have insulin resistance progressing to diabetes mellitus, while 80% of patients suffer from hypertension. They develop also distinctive physical features such as purple striae, easy bruising, and proximal muscle weakness. Patients with Cushing's syndrome due to either exogenous or endogenous cortisol excess exhibit several functional disorders that collectively comprise the metabolic syndrome phenotype [1, 22]. In addition to mentioned hypercortisolism manifestations, hypercortisolism (Cushing's syndrome) is usually associated with alterations in clotting and platelet function, as well as myocardial infarct size, and ventricular remodeling post-acute myocardial infarction [9]. These manifestations represent risk factors for cardiovascular diseases and demonstrate the systemic nature of cortisol excess.

The metabolic consequences of hypercortisolism extend beyond simple glucose intolerance to encompass the full spectrum of metabolic syndrome features, highlighting the central role of cortisol in metabolic homeostasis. Elevated cortisol provokes several physiological responses, including energy mobilization and homeostasis disturbance, therefore, implicating actions of cortisol different from its actions under normal circumstances.

5.3 Hypocortisolism and metabolic effects

Insufficient cortisol production (hypocortisolism) as seen in Addison's disease can lead to hypoglycemia, hypotension, electrolyte imbalances, and increased susceptibility to stress. This demonstrating the essential role of cortisol in maintaining metabolic homeostasis [36]. Addison's disease is characterized by attention deficit hyperactivity disorder and dyslexia, as well as circadian rhythm impairments, reflecting the importance of cortisol in neurocognitive function and temporal organization of physiological processes. Hypocortisolism results in impaired gluconeogenesis and decreased ability to maintain blood glucose during fasting or stress states. The inability to mount appropriate cortisol responses during physiological stress can result in life-threatening adrenal crises characterized by severe hypotension, dehydration, and electrolyte disturbances. In primary adrenal insufficiency, elevated ACTH levels may stimulate residual steroidogenic capacity, though this compensation is typically inadequate to maintain normal cortisol production [37]. The resulting metabolic phenotype includes enhanced insulin sensitivity due to the absence of cortisol's counter-regulatory effects, though this occurs at the expense of glucose homeostasis during stress states.

Recognition of hypocortisolism requires understanding of the metabolic consequences of cortisol deficiency and the need for physiological replacement therapy that mimics normal circadian cortisol patterns while providing additional coverage during stress states. This approach emphasizes the importance of maintaining both basal cortisol function and stress-responsive capacity for optimal metabolic health.

6. Conclusions

This comprehensive review of cortisol metabolism uncovers complex regulatory networks governing one of the body's most critical hormones. Cortisol's role extends far beyond its designation as a "stress hormone," encompassing essential functions in homeostasis of glucose, protein, and lipid. Cortisol is also considered as potent anti-inflammatory and immunosuppressant agent. Cortisol's actions are mediated through complex signaling pathways, while its regulation involves the precise interplay between the HPA axis, circadian rhythmicity, and tissue-specific enzymatic systems.

The clinical significance of cortisol metabolism is exemplified by the profound consequences of its dysregulation. Hypercortisolism causes cardiovascular complications and immune dysfunction, while hypocortisolism results in life-threatening metabolic instability and stress intolerance. These conditions emphasize the critical importance of maintaining appropriate cortisol levels and highlight the challenges inherent in therapeutic interventions targeting glucocorticoid pathways.

Sustained examination of cortisol metabolism will develop cortisol pharmacotherapy. The complexity of cortisol's actions across multiple physiological systems ensures ongoing opportunities for discovery new therapeutic interventions. Integration of basic science discoveries with clinical applications remains crucial for translating research advances into improved patient care. This making cortisol metabolism as a target for future innovations in endocrinology. As our understanding deepens, the goal remains to harness cortisol's beneficial effects while minimizing its potential for harm, ultimately leading to more effective and safer remedy for cortisol-related disorders.

Authors contributions

B.D.A. was responsible for chapter proposal and main concept; A.G.A. took care of chapter plan and design; B.D.A. and A.G.A. wrote, edited, and revised the first draft of the chapter; read the final version of the chapter; and agreed to submit it.

Funding

This scientific work received no external funding.

Conflict of interest

The authors declare no conflict of interest.

Author details

Abdulrahman G. Alharbi and Bandar D. Alrehaili*
Department of Pharmacology and Toxicology, College of Pharmacy, Taibah University, Medina, Kingdom of Saudi Arabia

*Address all correspondence to: brehaili@taibahu.edu.sa

References

[1] Wandja Vanessa K, Wankeu-Nya M, Murkwe M. Biological effects of cortisol. In: Păun DL, editor. Cortisol - between Physiology and Pathology [Internet]. Rijeka: IntechOpen; 2023. DOI: 10.5772/intechopen.1003161

[2] Chrousos GP. The hypothalamic–pituitary–adrenal axis and immune-mediated inflammation. New England Journal of Medicine [Internet]. 1995;**332**(20):1351-1363. DOI: 10.1056/NEJM199505183322008

[3] de Quervain DJF, Aerni A, Schelling G, Roozendaal B. Glucocorticoids and the regulation of memory in health and disease. Frontiers in Neuroendocrinology [Internet]. 2009;**30**(3):358-370. Available from: https://www.sciencedirect.com/science/article/pii/S009130220900003X

[4] Barsegyan A, Mackenzie SM, Kurose BD, McGaugh JL, Roozendaal B. Glucocorticoids in the prefrontal cortex enhance memory consolidation and impair working memory by a common neural mechanism. Proceedings of the National Academy of Sciences [Internet]. 2010;**107**(38):16655-16660. DOI: 10.1073/pnas.1011975107

[5] Knezevic E, Nenic K, Milanovic V, Knezevic NN. The role of cortisol in chronic stress, neurodegenerative diseases, and psychological disorders. Cells. 2023;**12**:2726. DOI: 10.3390/cells12232726

[6] Chrousos GP. Stress and disorders of the stress system. Nature Reviews Endocrinology [Internet]. 2009;**5**(7):374-381. DOI: 10.1038/nrendo.2009.106

[7] Erickson K, Drevets W, Schulkin J. Glucocorticoid regulation of diverse cognitive functions in normal and pathological emotional states. Neuroscience and Biobehavioral Reviews. 2003;**27**:233-246

[8] Elverson CA, Wilson ME. Cortisol: Circadian rhythm and response to a stressor. Newborn and Infant Nursing Reviews [Internet]. 2005;**5**(4):159-169. Available from: https://www.sciencedirect.com/science/article/pii/S1527336905001583

[9] Reincke M, Fleseriu M. Cushing syndrome: A review. JAMA. 2023;**330**:170-181

[10] Segerstrom SC, Miller GE. Psychological stress and the human immune system: A meta-analytic study of 30 years of inquiry NIH public access. Psychological Bulletin. 2004;**130**:601-630

[11] Vitlic A, Lord JM, Phillips AC. Stress, ageing and their influence on functional, cellular and molecular aspects of the immune system. Age. 2014;**36**:1169-1185

[12] Tasker JG, Dudek FE. Electrophysiological properties of neurones in the region of the paraventricular nucleus in slices of rat hypothalamus. Journal of Physiology. 1991;**434**:271-293

[13] Sheng JA, Bales NJ, Myers SA, Bautista AI, Roueinfar M, Hale TM, et al. The hypothalamic-pituitary-adrenal axis: Development, programming actions of hormones, and maternal-fetal interactions. Frontiers in Behavioral Neuroscience. 2021;**14**:601939. DOI: 10.3389/fnbeh.2020.601939

[14] Burford NG, Webster NA, Cruz-Topete D.

Hypothalamic-pituitary-adrenal axis modulation of glucocorticoids in the cardiovascular system. International Journal of Molecular Sciences. 2017;**18**

[15] Herman JP, McKlveen JM, Ghosal S, Kopp B, Wulsin A, Makinson R, et al. Regulation of the hypothalamic-pituitary- adrenocortical stress response. Comprehensive Physiology. 2016;**6**(2):603-621

[16] Miller WL. Disorders in the initial steps of steroid hormone synthesis. The Journal of Steroid Biochemistry and Molecular Biology [Internet]. 2017;**165**:18-37. Available from: https://www.sciencedirect.com/science/article/pii/S0960076016300553

[17] Manna PR, Dyson MT, Stocco DM. Regulation of the steroidogenic acute regulatory protein gene expression: Present and future perspectives. Molecular Human Reproduction. 2009;**15**:321-333

[18] Xie H, Su Y, Ge R. Steroidogenesis of corticosteroids, genetic mutation, and endocrine disruption leading to adrenal insufficiency. In: Păun DL, editor. Cortisol - between Physiology and Pathology [Internet]. Rijeka: IntechOpen; 2023. DOI: 10.5772/intechopen.1003273

[19] Yang M, White PC. Genetics and pathophysiology of classic congenital adrenal hyperplasia due to 21-hydroxylase deficiency. The Journal of Clinical Endocrinology & Metabolism [Internet]. 2025;**110**(Supplement_1):S1-S12. DOI: 10.1210/clinem/dgae535

[20] Ho MM, Vinson GP. 11β-hydroxylase gene expression in the rat adrenal cortex. Journal of Endocrinology [Internet]. 1993;**139**(2):301. Available from: https://joe.bioscientifica.com/view/journals/joe/139/2/joe_139_2_016.xml

[21] Kuo T, McQueen A, Chen TC, Wang JC. Regulation of glucose homeostasis by glucocorticoids. Advances in Experimental Medicine and Biology. 2015;**872**:99-126

[22] Thau L, Gandhi J, Sharma S. Physiology, Cortisol. In: StatPearls [Internet]. Treasure Island, FL: StatPearls Publishing; 2023. Available from: https://www.ncbi.nlm.nih.gov/sites/books/NBK538239/

[23] Han HS, Kang G, Kim JS, Choi BH, Koo SH. Regulation of glucose metabolism from a liver-centric perspective. Experimental and Molecular Medicine. 2016;**48**:e218-e218. DOI: 10.1038/emm.2015.122

[24] Peckett AJ, Wright DC, Riddell MC. The effects of glucocorticoids on adipose tissue lipid metabolism. Metabolism [Internet]. 2011;**60**(11):1500-1510. Available from: https://www.sciencedirect.com/science/article/pii/S0026049511001922

[25] Chai J, Wu Y, Sheng Z. The relationship between skeletal muscle proteolysis and ubiquitin–proteasome proteolytic pathway in burned rats. Burns [Internet]. 2002;**28**(6):527-533. Available from: https://www.sciencedirect.com/science/article/pii/S0305417902000499

[26] Kaplan SA, Shimizu CSN. Effects of cortisol on amino acids in skeletal muscle and plasma. Endocrinology [Internet]. 1963;**72**(2):267-272. DOI: 10.1210/endo-72-2-267

[27] Hue L, Taegtmeyer H. The Randle cycle revisited: A new head for an old hat. American Journal of Physiology - Endocrinology and

Metabolism. 2009;**297**:E578-E591. DOI: 10.1152/ajpendo.00093.2009

[28] Debono M, Prema A, Hughes TJB, Bull M, Ross RJ, Newell-Price J. Visceral fat accumulation and postdexamethasone serum cortisol levels in patients with adrenal incidentaloma. The Journal of Clinical Endocrinology & Metabolism [Internet]. 2013;**98**(6):2383-2391. DOI: 10.1210/jc.2012-4276

[29] Lindroos J, Husa J, Mitterer G, Haschemi A, Rauscher S, Haas R, et al. Human but not mouse adipogenesis is critically dependent on LMO3. Cell Metabolism. 2013;**18**(1):62-74

[30] Mccarthy TL, Cenrella M, Canalis E. Cortisol inhibits the synthesis of insulin-like growth factor-I in skeletal cells. Endocrinology [Internet]. 1990;**126**(3):1569-1575. DOI: 10.1210/endo-126-3-1569

[31] Rhyu J, Yu R. Newly discovered endocrine functions of the liver. World Journal of Hepatology. 2021;**13**(11):1611-1628

[32] Gambineri A, Forlani G, Munarini A, Tomassoni F, Cognigni GE, Ciampaglia W, et al. Increased clearance of cortisol by 5β-reductase in a subgroup of women with adrenal hyperandrogenism in polycystic ovary syndrome. Journal of Endocrinological Investigation. 2009;**32**:210-218. DOI: 10.1007/BF03346454

[33] Chapman K, Holmes M, Seckl J. 11β-hydroxysteroid dehydrogenases intracellular gate-keepers of tissue glucocorticoid action. Physiological Reviews. 2013;**93**(3):1139-1206

[34] Kataoka S, Kudo A, Hirano H, Kawakami H, Kawano T, Higashihara E, et al. 11β-hydroxysteroid dehydrogenase type 2 is expressed in the human kidney glomerulus. The Journal of Clinical Endocrinology & Metabolism. 2002;**87**(2):877-882. DOI: 10.1210/jcem.87.2.8257

[35] Bonnet-Serrano F, Nakib S, Zientek C, Guignat L, Guibourdenche J, Bertherat J, et al. Urinary free cortisol determination and interferences studies using liquid chromatography coupled to tandem mass spectrometry after on-line solid phase extraction based on Turboflow™ chromatography. Metabolites. 2023;**13**(10):1063. DOI: 10.3390/metabo13101063

[36] Raymond GV, Moser AB, Fatemi A. X-Linked Adrenoleukodystrophy Synonym: X-ALD. In Gene Reviews [Internet]. Seattle (WA): University of Washington; 1999. Available from: https://www.ncbi.nlm.nih.gov/books/NBK1315/

[37] Alexandraki KI, Sanpawithayakul K, Grossman A. Adrenal Insufficiency. In: Endotext [Internet]. South Dartmouth (MA): MDText.com, Inc.; 2022. Available from: https://europepmc.org/article/nbk/nbk279083

Section 2

HPA Axis Testing and Corticosteroid Therapy in Clinical Practice

Chapter 4

Laboratory Evaluation of the Hypothalamic-Pituitary-Adrenal Axis

Daniela Greere and Diana Loreta Păun

Abstract

Diagnosis of endocrine disorders often requires a high index of suspicion, thorough clinical assessment and adequate laboratory analysis. Cortisol is a vital steroid hormone involved in stress response, regulating blood pressure, metabolism and circadian rhythm, inflammatory response, and immune function. Laboratory evaluation of the hypothalamic-pituitary-adrenal (HPA) axis is essential for diagnosing disorders of cortisol production, including differentiating between primary adrenal insufficiency (Addison's disease) and secondary adrenal insufficiency, and assessing hypercortisolism (including Cushing syndrome). This chapter provides a comprehensive overview of the main laboratory tests used to evaluate the HPA axis function, namely basal hormone measurements and dynamic stimulation or suppression tests. It emphasizes the clinical interpretation of test results in various pathological contexts, highlighting factors that may interfere with assay accuracy and physiological variability. Practical considerations regarding the integration of biochemical findings with clinical data are also discussed. Ultimately, the chapter aims to guide clinicians and laboratory specialists in selecting, performing, and interpreting appropriate tests to ensure accurate diagnosis and effective management of HPA axis disorders.

Keywords: hypothalamo-hypophyseal system, pituitary-adrenal system, cortisol, adrenal insufficiency, Cushing syndrome, adrenocorticotropic hormone, dexamethasone suppression test, ACTH stimulation test

1. Introduction

Diagnosis of endocrine disorders often requires a high index of suspicion, thorough clinical assessment and adequate laboratory analysis. Cortisol is a vital steroid hormone involved in stress response, regulating blood pressure, metabolism and circadian rhythm, inflammatory response, and immune function. Laboratory evaluation of the hypothalamic-pituitary-adrenal (HPA) axis is essential for diagnosing disorders of cortisol production, including differentiating between primary and secondary adrenal insufficiency, and assessing hypercortisolism [1].

1.1 Brief physiology refresher

The hypothalamic-pituitary-adrenal (HPA) axis is a key neuroendocrine system regulating multiple homeostatic processes, including metabolism, immune function, and cardiovascular stability, as well as the stress response. Neurons in the hypothalamic paraventricular nucleus produce corticotropin-releasing hormone (CRH), which travels *via* the hypophyseal portal system to the anterior pituitary, stimulating adrenocorticotropic hormone (ACTH) secretion. Arginine vasopressin (AVP) also acts as a co-secretagogue [1].

CRH stimulates the transcription of the POMC (proopiomelanocortin) gene, which encodes a large precursor protein. This precursor undergoes post-translational modification in secretory granules, where enzymes cleave it into several biologically active peptides, including ACTH (a 39-amino acid N-terminal fragment) and alpha-melanocyte-stimulating hormone (α-MSH).

ACTH enters systemic circulation, binds to melanocortin 2 receptors in the adrenal cortex, and thus prompts the adrenal cortex to produce cortisol and weak androgens, such as dehydroepiandrosterone sulfate (DHEA-S). Cortisol then inhibits further CRH and ACTH release through negative feedback, thereby regulating its own levels and the stress response [1].

ACTH and cortisol secretion follow a circadian rhythm, peaking in the early morning and reaching their lowest levels (nadir) around midnight. Under normal conditions, only 5–10% of circulating cortisol is free and biologically active. About 85% binds to cortisol-binding globulin (CBG), and 5–10% binds to albumin, which has low affinity, making the albumin-bound fraction also available. Unbound cortisol is filtered by the kidneys and subsequently excreted in urine. Urinary cortisol reflects free, circulating cortisol levels in the blood [1].

1.2 Clinical evaluation

The physical examination and medical history should focus on identifying clinical features suggestive of cortisol deficiency or excess, as well as factors that may interfere with tests' accuracy, including concomitant medications, alterations in dexamethasone metabolism, night-shift work, abnormal cortisol-binding globulin levels, and coexisting sleep disorders [2].

Primary adrenal insufficiency (Addison disease) results from destruction or dysfunction of the adrenal cortex and is characterized by fatigue, weight loss, anorexia, hypotension (which initially manifests as orthostatic hypotension and in adrenal crisis setting manifests as vasodilatory shock) and gastrointestinal symptoms (nausea, vomiting, diarrhea, abdominal pain). A distinguishing feature is hyperpigmentation of the skin and mucosa, caused by the elevated ACTH and α-MSH levels. Laboratory findings often include hyponatremia, hyperkalemia, and salt craving due to mineralocorticoid deficiency. Causes of primary adrenal insufficiency include autoimmune Addison's disease (the most common etiology in adults), as well as genetic and congenital disorders such as congenital adrenal hyperplasia, familial glucocorticoid deficiency, and rarer multisystem conditions (e.g., sphingolipid metabolism disorders such as SGPL1 deficiency), which are more commonly seen in pediatric or early-onset cases [1].

In contrast, central (secondary or tertiary) adrenal insufficiency is caused by pituitary or hypothalamic disorders or by chronic glucocorticoid therapy. Patients may present with fatigue, weakness, and hypotension, but hyperpigmentation and hyperkalemia are absent since mineralocorticoid secretion is preserved [1].

Cushing syndrome results from chronic excess glucocorticoid exposure and is characterized by progressive weight gain with faciotruncal fat distribution (central obesity, facial rounding "moon face," dorsocervical fat accumulation "buffalo hump"), and manifestations of protein catabolism (skin thinning with easy bruising and purple striae, proximal muscle weakness). Metabolic and systemic consequences frequently include arterial hypertension, glucose intolerance or diabetes, osteoporosis, hypogonadism, and neuropsychiatric symptoms (most often depression, anxiety, insomnia, and cognitive impairment). From a clinical perspective, it is important to note that when glucocorticoid excess is accompanied by androgen excess, the typical manifestations of protein catabolism may be absent or less pronounced. Furthermore, unlike the gradual onset of Cushing disease (ACTH-producing pituitary adenoma), paraneoplastic Cushing syndrome (ectopic ACTH secretion) usually develops rapidly, with the clinical picture dominated by the catabolic effects of severe cortisol excess (including marked muscle wasting and weakness), and significant hypokalemia. Recognition of these characteristic clinical features provides an essential framework for selecting appropriate biochemical tests to evaluate the hypothalamic-pituitary-adrenal axis [1].

2. Adrenal insufficiency

2.1 Indications for evaluation

Clinical manifestations of adrenal insufficiency (AI) vary by onset. Acute AI can present as adrenal crisis, while chronic forms often have subtle, nonspecific symptoms (orthostatic hypotension, and weight-loss and non-specific gastrointestinal symptoms, such as nausea, vomiting, diarrhea, abdominal pain), necessitating high clinical suspicion for diagnosis. Low basal morning serum cortisol (within 3 hours of awakening, typically 6–9 AM) may suggest AI but is insufficient for definitive diagnosis; dynamic stimulation tests are essential when baseline results are inconclusive. **Table 1** comprises a summary of the main baseline and dynamic hormonal tests used in the diagnosis of AI.

Testing is indicated in adults with relevant clinical features or risk factors [3–5]:

- Adrenal crisis: Consider AI in any patient with vasodilatory shock, regardless of prior history.
- Chronic AI: Suspect in patients with fatigue, weakness, myalgias, arthralgias, anorexia, weight loss, and hyponatremia. Hyperkalemia, salt craving, and hyperpigmentation are specific to primary AI. Postural hypotension is common in primary and can occur acutely in central AI. Isolated ACTH deficiency, though rare, should be considered in unexplained severe hypoglycemia or hyponatremia.
- Chronic glucocorticoid therapy: Assess for AI before discontinuing or rapidly reducing glucocorticoids, especially after >3 weeks of therapy. Gradual tapering is advised. Early-morning cortisol (8–9 AM), 24 hours after last dose, helps assess adrenal function. Indeterminate results (5–<10 mcg/dL) may require ACTH stimulation testing.

Test	Indication/ purpose	Principle/what it assesses	Brief interpretation
Morning serum cortisol (6–9 AM)	Suspected chronic adrenal insufficiency	Measures basal cortisol near peak circadian secretion	≤3 μg/dL confirms AI; >3–<18 μg/dL indeterminate → ACTH test; ≥18 μg/dL excludes AI
Random cortisol in suspected adrenal crisis	Hemodynamic instability/shock	Assesses acute cortisol reserve	<18 μg/dL in hypotension suggests adrenal crisis; ≥18 μg/dL makes AI unlikely
ACTH stimulation test (250 μg, high-dose)	Indeterminate morning cortisol; suspected primary/ secondary AI	Synthetic ACTH stimulates adrenal cortisol secretion	Peak ≥18 μg/dL (or ≥ 14–15 μg/dL LC-MS/MS) excludes AI; <14 μg/dL suggests AI
Low-dose ACTH test (1 μg)	Historically subtle central AI (no longer recommended)	Physiologic ACTH dose tests adrenal sensitivity	Blunted cortisol rise suggests AI; limited utility and dilution errors
DHEA-S	Adjunct to differentiate AI likelihood	Adrenal androgen production regulated by ACTH	Normal DHEAS makes AI unlikely; low DHEAS supportive, but not diagnostic
17-Hydroxyprogesterone ± cosyntropin (CAH Testing)	Suspected congenital adrenal hyperplasia	Evaluates steroid precursor accumulation before/after ACTH	Baseline or stimulated 17-OHP above diagnostic cutoffs confirms CAH
Insulin tolerance test (ITT)	Gold standard for secondary/central AI; post-pituitary surgery evaluation	Hypoglycemia stimulates CRH → ACTH → cortisol	Peak ≥18 μg/dL (or ≥ 14–15 μg/dL LC-MS/MS) excludes AI; <14 μg/dL suggests AI
Overnight metyrapone test	Detection of partial ACTH deficiency/ secondary AI	Blocks cortisol synthesis → ACTH rise → ↑11-deoxycortisol	11-deoxycortisol 7–22 μg/dL + cortisol <5–7 mcg/dL,= normal; 11-deoxycortisol<7 mcg/dL + cortisol <5–7 mcg/dL, ACTH deficiency
CBG measurement	Clarify discordant cortisol values	Measures cortisol-binding globulin affecting total cortisol	High CBG → falsely high cortisol; low CBG → falsely low cortisol
Renin and aldosterone	Differentiate primary vs. secondary adrenal insufficiency	Assesses mineralocorticoid axis integrity	High renin + low aldosterone, primary AI; normal values, secondary AI

ACTH, adrenocorticotropic hormone; AI, adrenal insufficiency; CAH, congenital adrenal hyperplasia; CBG, corticosteroid-binding globulin; DHEA-S, dehydroepiandrosterone sulfate; LC-MS/MS, liquid chromatography–tandem mass spectrometry.

Table 1.
The main baseline and dynamic hormonal tests used in the diagnosis of adrenal insufficiency.

Nota bene: Although individual susceptibility varies, current evidence suggests that the risk of clinically significant HPA-axis suppression is generally low after a single short glucocorticoid course of less than 3–4 weeks; risk increases with repeated courses, longer duration, higher potency, and interacting medications.

- Perioperative glucocorticoid therapy: Chronic glucocorticoid use may blunt the adrenal stress response during surgery. Routine HPA axis assessment is not needed if therapy continues perioperatively.

- Congenital adrenal hyperplasia (CAH): An autosomal recessive disorder, most commonly due to 21-hydroxylase deficiency (95% of cases). Screening uses 17-hydroxyprogesterone (17-OHP); ACTH stimulation confirms diagnosis and assesses cortisol production in non-classical CAH, guiding stress-dose corticosteroid needs.

The diagnostic approach for adrenal insufficiency involves three key steps: first, excluding functional or medication-induced (exogenous) suppression of the hypothalamic-pituitary-adrenal (HPA) axis; second, confirming the presence of true adrenal insufficiency through clinical assessment and biochemical testing (such as morning serum cortisol, ACTH, and dynamic stimulation tests); and third, determining the underlying etiology—distinguishing between primary (adrenal), secondary, or tertiary (central) causes—using additional hormonal measurements and targeted imaging. In patients with persistent clinical suspicion but inconclusive or borderline test results, repeat evaluation and dynamic testing are recommended, as delayed or missed diagnosis of adrenal insufficiency can lead to life-threatening complications.

2.2 Hormonal assessment

Basal cortisol measurement is not diagnostic for adrenal insufficiency (AI), but can help exclude AI or identify patients needing further evaluation [6]. Due to the broad reference range of morning cortisol and the pulsatile secretion pattern, some individuals with AI may show normal ACTH or cortisol levels. Therefore, a single morning cortisol result may be inconclusive. When baseline cortisol is indeterminate or clinical findings do not match laboratory results, dynamic stimulation testing is necessary to confirm or exclude AI.

Suspected adrenal crisis: Obtain serum ACTH and cortisol immediately after IV access is established, but do not delay treatment for results. A cortisol level below 18 mcg/dL (<500 nmol/L) in hypotensive patients suggests adrenal insufficiency; diagnosis should be confirmed with an ACTH stimulation test later. A basal cortisol ≥18 mcg/dL (≥500 nmol/L) makes adrenal insufficiency unlikely.

Suspected chronic adrenal insufficiency: Measure serum cortisol within 3 hours of awakening (6–9 AM) in individuals with suspected chronic adrenal insufficiency. When primary adrenal insufficiency is strongly suspected (e.g., orthostatic hypotension with hyperpigmentation, hyponatremia, hyperkalemia), assess serum cortisol, plasma ACTH, renin, and aldosterone concurrently. Early primary adrenal insufficiency may present with decreased aldosterone and increased renin prior to overt cortisol deficiency [3]. Interpretation: An early morning serum cortisol ≤3 mcg/dL (80 nmol/L), excluding corticosteroid-binding globulin (CBG) deficiency, confirms adrenal insufficiency [7]. If clinical features align, ACTH stimulation testing is generally unnecessary. If there is a mismatch between clinical and biochemical findings, ACTH stimulation testing is needed, as some patients with low morning cortisol may respond normally. For morning cortisol >3 mcg/dL but <18 mcg/dL (or 14–15 mcg/dL by liquid chromatography tandem mass spectrometry LC-MS/MS), perform an ACTH stimulation test. A value ≥18 mcg/dL (≥500 nmol/L) effectively excludes adrenal insufficiency if CBG is not elevated [3].

Congenital adrenal hyperplasia: A comprehensive adrenal steroid profile—including 17-OHP, progesterone, cortisol, DOC, 11-deoxycortisol, pregnenolone, 17-hydroxypregnenolone, DHEA, and androstenedione—should be obtained before and 60 minutes after 250 mcg of cosyntropin. Per the 2018 Endocrine Society Guideline, cosyntropin stimulation testing is recommended if 17-hydroxyprogesterone (17-OHP) is indeterminate or if alternative enzyme deficiencies (such as 11β-hydroxylase, 3β-hydroxysteroid dehydrogenase type 2, 17α-hydroxylase, or P450 oxidoreductase) are suspected. Basal or stimulated 17-OHP >1000 ng/dL (30 nmol/L) confirms CAH [5]. Recent updates indicate that 17-OHP >7–10 ng/mL by immunoassay or > 3 ng/mL by LC-MS/MS, at baseline or after stimulation, are diagnostic [8]. For more details, see: [9].

DHEA-S: Measurement of DHEAS can aid in evaluating suspected adrenal insufficiency. A normal DHEAS (using age- and sex-specific reference ranges) makes adrenal insufficiency unlikely, while reduced DHEAS levels are typically seen in both primary and central adrenal insufficiencies [10]. When combined with early morning cortisol measurements, diagnostic accuracy improves, and ACTH stimulation testing may sometimes be avoided. For example, most patients with baseline cortisol <5 mcg/dL and DHEAS <25 mcg/dL were confirmed to have adrenal insufficiency [11]. However, low DHEAS alone is not diagnostic; if cortisol values are indeterminate and DHEAS is low or equivocal, ACTH stimulation testing is still required.

Standard high-dose ACTH stimulation test. The standard high-dose (250 mcg) ACTH stimulation test is essential for diagnosing adrenal insufficiency in patients with indeterminate basal cortisol and clinical suspicion of hypoadrenalism. This test uses synthetic ACTH (1–24) (cosyntropin), which stimulates the adrenal cortex *via* the MC2R receptor, inducing cortisol release. The 250 mcg dose creates supraphysiologic ACTH levels, assessing the adrenal gland's maximal cortisol output. Impaired cortisol response indicates primary adrenal insufficiency or adrenal atrophy from chronic ACTH deficiency. However, in recent-onset ACTH deficiency (e.g., within 4–6 weeks of pituitary surgery or radiotherapy), the test may yield a falsely normal result before adrenal atrophy occurs; in such cases, alternative tests like insulin-induced hypoglycemia or metyrapone testing may be required [12].

Procedure: The standard high-dose ACTH stimulation test can be performed at any time of day. Glucocorticoids should be withheld on the morning of the test and resumed afterward. After obtaining a baseline serum cortisol sample, administer 250 mcg cosyntropin intramuscularly or intravenously (diluted in 2–5 mL saline over 2 minutes for IV use). Collect serum cortisol at 30 and 60 minutes post-injection. Interpretation: Cortisol responses are best assessed by absolute thresholds rather than increments. The highest cortisol value post-stimulation is used for interpretation:

- Serum cortisol <14 mcg/dL (390 nmol/L) strongly suggests adrenal insufficiency.
- Values between 14 and 18 mcg/dL (390–500 nmol/L) require consideration of assay type and clinical context; with LC-MS/MS, the upper threshold is 14–15 mcg/dL [13]. In uncertain cases, a normal age- and sex-adjusted DHEAS supports normal adrenal function.
- Serum cortisol ≥18 mcg/dL (≥500 nmol/L) generally excludes adrenal insufficiency.

Contraindications: Cosyntropin is contraindicated in patients with known hypersensitivity to the drug or its excipients (e.g., mannitol) and should be used cautiously in individuals with pre-existing allergic conditions.

Adverse reactions: The ACTH stimulation test is generally safe, with the adverse effects being rare and usually mild. Reported reactions (1–10%) include flushing, low-grade fever, pruritus, and, rarely, gastrointestinal symptoms such as nausea, vomiting, and abdominal pain. Hypersensitivity reactions occur in less than 1% of cases.

Clinical application and additional considerations

- In hemodynamically unstable patients, initiate IV crystalloid resuscitation and administer dexamethasone before testing if primary adrenal insufficiency is suspected.

- The ACTH stimulation test may yield falsely normal results if performed within 4–6 weeks of hypothalamic or pituitary injury (e.g., post-surgery).

- Abnormal corticosteroid-binding globulin (CBG) levels can confound test results: High CBG (e.g., pregnancy, oral contraceptives, estrogen therapy) may falsely elevate cortisol; low CBG (e.g., nephrotic syndrome, severe illness) may lower cortisol readings. Measuring CBG is helpful when results are unexpected.

- Clinical guidelines recommend discontinuing oral estrogen therapy 1.5–3 months before adrenal testing [3]. Transdermal estrogen has minimal impact and usually does not require discontinuation [14].

- In case of low albumin (<2.5 g/dL) or low CBG measurement of free cortisol is preferred (normal peak >1.2 μg/dL at 30 or 60 minutes) [15].

- Early primary adrenal insufficiency may present with low aldosterone and elevated renin before overt cortisol deficiency and ACTH elevation.

- For assessment of baseline ACTH, renin, DHEAS, and aldosterone, testing should occur between 6 and 9 AM or within 4 hours of awakening to minimize diurnal variation. Baseline electrolyte and plasma renin measurements aid interpretation of aldosterone values. In primary adrenal insufficiency, all adrenal zones are affected, causing hyponatremia, hyperkalemia, low aldosterone, and elevated renin. Central adrenal insufficiency typically spares the renin-angiotensin system, resulting in normal potassium, renin, and aldosterone, with possible hyponatremia due to other mechanisms. Aldosterone can also be measured at 30- and 60-minute post-ACTH, as ACTH stimulates its secretion; in healthy individuals, aldosterone rises by roughly 190% after 250 mcg ACTH [16]. A normal aldosterone response with suboptimal cortisol suggests secondary adrenal insufficiency.

- Critical illness: Critically ill patients have reduced cortisol clearance, resulting in variable cortisol and ACTH levels. Definitions of normal cortisol during critical illness are unclear, and binding globulin abnormalities are common, making lab assays unreliable [17]. Glucocorticoid therapy decisions in septic shock are generally based on clinical judgment rather than lab testing.

Low dose ACTH stimulation test (1 mcg ACTH). The low-dose ACTH stimulation test was developed to increase sensitivity for detecting secondary adrenal insufficiency by using a more physiologic ACTH dose. However, this test is not recommended in current clinical practice and should not be used routinely. It does not provide a clear diagnostic advantage over the standard high-dose test. Additionally, commercial low-dose cosyntropin preparations are unavailable, and accurate dilution and administration of ACTH(1-24) are impractical.

The insulin tolerance test (ITT). The insulin-induced hypoglycemia test assesses adrenal function by provoking hypoglycemia, which triggers CRH, ACTH, and ultimately cortisol release. ITT is considered the gold standard for diagnosing secondary adrenal insufficiency. However, because of its complexity, higher risk, and cost, it is rarely used in routine practice. Its primary indication is after recent pituitary surgery, when the ACTH stimulation test may give falsely normal results during the initial 1–2 months [18].

Procedure: For the insulin tolerance test (ITT), patients fast for at least 8 hours and remain supine throughout. Continuous medical supervision is required due to the risk of hypoglycemia-related complications, such as chest pain, tachycardia, confusion, or seizures. A syringe with 50% glucose should be readily available. After establishing IV access, regular insulin is administered IV at 0.15 units/kg (adjusted to 0.2 units/kg for those with obesity, diabetes, acromegaly, or Cushing syndrome, and 0.1 units/kg for suspected hypopituitarism or primary adrenal insufficiency). Blood samples for bedside glucose, serum glucose, and cortisol are taken before insulin and every 15 minutes afterward; ACTH may be measured if indicated. The key sample for ACTH and cortisol is collected 5–10 minutes after diaphoresis onset or when serum glucose drops below 35 mg/dL (1.9 mmol/L), though some protocols use higher thresholds. If adequate hypoglycemia is not achieved, a second insulin dose is given, which usually induces the target hypoglycemia within an additional 30 to 45 minutes. After the test, patients receive sweetened fluids (orange juice or cola) and glucose is monitored at 5 , 10 and 15 minutes after feeding. If symptoms persist or are severe, administer 25 g of 50% glucose IV slowly, over the course of 1 minute (this leads to hyperglycemia within 30 seconds). Cortisol samples should also be obtained at the time of glucose administration and 15 minutes later, as cortisol may continue to rise post-hypoglycemia [19]. Interpretation of the ITT is based on the peak serum cortisol value, similar to the standard high-dose ACTH test [19]. With older assays, normal responses range from 18 to 22 mcg/dL (500–600 nmol/L), but newer immunoassays and LC-MS/MS yield results up to 25% lower; thus, cortisol cutoffs must be assay-specific [13]. A peak plasma ACTH above 150 pg./mL (33 pmol/L) is generally considered normal, though precise reference values are not established [20]. Salivary cortisol measurement during ITT shows promise for diagnosis, but specific cutoffs remain undefined [21].

Contraindications—This test is contraindicated in patients with coronary heart disease, cerebrovascular disease, or epilepsy because the acute hypoglycemia produced during the test can trigger significant physiological stress responses. In patients with coronary heart disease, hypoglycemia activates the sympathoadrenal system, leading to tachycardia, increased blood pressure, and elevated myocardial oxygen demand, which may precipitate myocardial ischemia or arrhythmias. In individuals with cerebrovascular disease, severe hypoglycemia may compromise cerebral perfusion and increase the risk of transient ischemic attacks or stroke. Similarly, hypoglycemia lowers the seizure threshold, making the test potentially dangerous in patients with epilepsy, as it can provoke generalized seizures. For these reasons, safer alternative dynamic tests, such as the ACTH stimulation test, are generally preferred in these populations.

Special considerations:

- The ITT can be performed at any time, but morning testing is preferred due to fasting requirements.
- Hydrocortisone or cortisone acetate should be withheld for at least 12 hours before the test, if possible.
- The ITT should not be done while the patient is taking dexamethasone, as it suppresses the necessary hypothalamic response.
- Hypoglycemia is a stronger stimulus for ACTH secretion than metyrapone-induced hypocortisolemia, so the ITT may miss partial adrenal insufficiency detected by the metyrapone test; rarely, the reverse occurs [22].
- The ITT combined with CRH stimulation test can help distinguish hypothalamic from pituitary dysfunction. If the ITT fails to elicit a cortisol response, but the CRH stimulation test produces an appropriate increase in cortisol, this pattern suggests that the dysfunction is localized to the hypothalamus. The CRH test is now rarely used due to limited availability.
- Growth hormone (GH) can also be assessed during ITT; however, diagnostic cutoffs vary considerably depending on assay methodology, geographic practice, and specialist center, with commonly used thresholds ranging from approximately 3 to 10 mcg/L. A peak GH value ≤5 mcg/L is frequently cited as a reference cutoff for adult GH deficiency, although lower thresholds may be more appropriate in individuals with obesity [23]. However, alternative dynamic tests for GH deficiency (such as the arginine-GHRH test, the macimorelin test, and the glucagon stimulation test) have largely replaced ITT for this purpose [24].

The overnight single-dose metyrapone test. The metyrapone stimulation test assesses adrenal function by inhibiting the conversion of 11-deoxycortisol to cortisol. As 11-deoxycortisol lacks significant glucocorticoid activity, decreased cortisol levels trigger increased ACTH secretion and accumulation of 11-deoxycortisol. A blunted or absent rise in ACTH or 11-deoxycortisol suggests ACTH deficiency or primary adrenal disease, requiring further evaluation. The overnight metyrapone test, performed 6 weeks after transsphenoidal surgery, correlates well with the insulin tolerance test but carries fewer risks, making it preferable when available [25]. It is mainly used to detect partial defects in pituitary ACTH secretion and can be conducted in an outpatient setting [26].

Procedure: Metyrapone is given orally at 30 mg/kg or as a fixed dose (2 g if <70 kg, 2.5 g if 70–90 kg, 3 g if >90 kg) at midnight with a glass of milk or snack. Serum 11-deoxycortisol and cortisol are measured the next morning (7:30–9:30 AM); plasma ACTH may also be assessed for additional information [27]. Interpretation: A normal response is a morning 11-deoxycortisol level of 7–22 mcg/dL (200–635 nmol/L) with a simultaneous cortisol <5–7 mcg/dL (138–193 nmol/L), confirming adequate metyrapone effect and compliance. A level of 11-deoxycortisol <7 mcg/dL (202 nmol/L) with suppressed cortisol indicates adrenal insufficiency. A higher cutoff (e.g., 10 mcg/dL, 276 nmol/L) may improve diagnostic accuracy in those with moderate-to-low pretest probability of secondary adrenal insufficiency [26].

Caveats in interpretation:

- False-negative results may occur when 11-deoxycortisol rises excessively, as seen in hypothyroidism, hypoglycemia, diabetes, heart failure, obesity, or chronic kidney disease. Assess thyroid function before testing [28].

- False-positives can result from recent high-dose glucocorticoid use, which suppresses corticotrope function, or from rapid metyrapone clearance, leading to inadequate cortisol suppression (cortisol >7.5 mcg/dL at 8 AM); this occurs in about 4% of healthy subjects. Medications that induce hepatic CYP450 (e.g., phenobarbital, phenytoin, rifampin, mitotane) should be stopped well before testing [28].

- Estrogens and oral contraceptives can artificially elevate 11-deoxycortisol due to effects on corticosteroid-binding globulin.

- Some cortisol immunoassays cross-react with 11-deoxycortisol, causing falsely high cortisol readings. Use highly specific immunoassays or LC-MS/MS for accurate measurement.

Metyrapone side effects: Metyrapone can trigger adrenal insufficiency symptoms—such as hypotension, nausea, vomiting, abdominal pain, and muscle aches—especially in those with underlying adrenal insufficiency. Other side effects include dizziness, sedation, allergic rash, and rarely, leukopenia or bone marrow suppression. The test should not be performed outpatient if severe adrenal insufficiency is suspected. If symptoms develop during testing, administer 10 mg hydrocortisone after sample collection and before discharge.

An inadequate cortisol response to the aforementioned stimulation tests is indicative of adrenal insufficiency of any cause. Determining the pathophysiological form requires interpretation of morning ACTH levels. It is important to note that ACTH is heat labile; improper handling or failure to keep samples on ice can result in proteolysis and falsely low ACTH concentrations. In cases of primary adrenal insufficiency, plasma ACTH concentrations are typically 5–10 times above the upper limit of normal (often exceeding 100 pg./mL), with elevated renin and reduced aldosterone and DHEA-S levels [29]. These patients typically exhibit dehydration, hyperkalemia, and skin hyperpigmentation. In contrast, secondary adrenal insufficiency is characterized by low or inappropriately normal ACTH levels, low DHEA-S, with renin and aldosterone values within the reference range. These patients are more likely to experience hypoglycemia, but do not exhibit dehydration, hyperkalemia, or skin hyperpigmentation.

Establishing the underlying etiology necessitates a comprehensive approach, including detailed patient history, clinical examination, imaging studies (such as abdominal computed tomography for evaluation of the adrenal glands and magnetic resonance imaging of the pituitary and hypothalamus), and laboratory investigations. These may comprise testing for anti-adrenal antibodies (21-hydroxylase autoantibodies, indicative of autoimmunity), as well as screening for infectious etiologies (such as HIV or tuberculosis) and genetic disorders.

3. Hypercortisolism and Cushing syndrome

3.1 Indications for evaluation

Hypercortisolism (HCM) describes excessive tissue exposure to cortisol or related glucocorticoids, from either endogenous or exogenous sources. When persistent and pathological, this leads to Cushing syndrome (CS), characterized by a distinct set of clinical and laboratory findings. Other forms—including subclinical CS, iatrogenic/exogenous CS, cyclical CS, and pseudo-CS (physiologic HCM)—are more common than classic CS and are often harder to diagnose and manage [30]. Diagnostic tests for CS typically evaluate 24-hour cortisol secretion, adherence to the normal circadian rhythm, and the integrity of the negative feedback mechanism. In endogenous CS, cortisol production is increased, circadian rhythm is lost, and the HPA axis shows resistance to feedback inhibition. Endogenous CS is further classified as ACTH-dependent or ACTH-independent [31].

Screening for Cushing syndrome is recommended for young adults with osteoporosis, early-onset hypertension, or hyperglycemia/diabetes; individuals of any age with unexplained severe diseases such as resistant hypertension or osteoporosis; patients with progressive or characteristic signs of hypercortisolism (facial plethora, proximal myopathy, easy bruising, or wide pigmented striae); and those with adrenal incidentalomas [32]. Acute physical or emotional stress activates the HPA axis, leading to the elevated ACTH and cortisol levels. Therefore, the assessment for Cushing syndrome should be postponed until after acute stress has resolved. **Table 2** comprises a summary of the main baseline and dynamic hormonal tests used in the diagnosis of Cushing's syndrome.

Test	Indication/purpose	Principle/what it assesses	Brief interpretation
24-hour urinary free cortisol (UFC)	First-line screening; preferred in pregnancy, altered CBG, cyclic CS.	Measures total free cortisol secretion over 24 h.	≥3× ULN twice or one sample ≥ 3× ULN + another abnormal screening test, CS. Mild elevation → pseudo-Cushing possible.
Late-night salivary cortisol	First-line screening; preferred in altered CBG, pregnancy, cyclic CS.	Assesses loss of cortisol circadian nadir.	Two elevated samples or one elevated sample + another abnormal screening test = CS.
Late-night serum cortisol	Inpatient alternative to late-night salivary cortisol	Assesses loss of cortisol circadian nadir.	>7.5 mcg/dL suggests CS; Two elevated samples or one elevated sample + another abnormal screening test = CS
1-mg Overnight DST	First-line screening or confirmatory test for endogenous CS; adrenal incidentaloma evaluation.	Assess HPA feedback suppression.	<1.8 mcg/dL excludes CS; lack of suppression indicates CS.
2-day Low-dose DST	Alternative confirmatory test for endogenous CS.	Assess HPA feedback suppression.	<1.8 mcg/dL excludes CS; lack of suppression indicates CS.
High-dose DST (HDDST)	Differentiate ACTH-dependent causes: pituitary vs. ectopic.	Pituitary tumors partially suppress with high-dose dex.	>50% cortisol suppression → Cushing disease. No suppression does not exclude CD.

Test	Indication/purpose	Principle/what it assesses	Brief interpretation
Dexamethasone–CRH Test	Differentiate pseudo-Cushing vs. Cushing disease (CD).	CRH overcomes dex suppression only in CD.	Cortisol >1.4 mcg/dL at 15 min suggests Cushing disease.
Desmopressin Test	Supports diagnosis of Cushing disease.	ACTH-secreting pituitary tumors respond to DDAVP.	≥20% cortisol + ≥50% ACTH rise suggests CD. False positives possible.
Bilateral inferior petrosal sinus sampling (BIPSS)	Gold standard to localize ACTH source.	Measures central-to-peripheral (C:P) ACTH gradient.	CD: with CRH, C:P > 2 baseline or > 3 post-stim; with DDAVP, >1.4 baseline, >2.8 post-stim.
Serum ACTH	Differentiate ACTH-dependent vs. independent CS.	Measures ACTH drive.	<5 pg./mL, ACTH-independent; >20 pg./mL, ACTH-dependent; 5–20 pg./mL, dynamic tests needed.
Serum DHEA-S	Adjunct for ACTH dependence.	Reflects chronic ACTH stimulation.	Low, ACTH-independent; normal/high, ACTH-dependent.
Adrenal vein sampling (AVS)	Indicated in ACTH-independent Cushing's syndrome with bilateral adrenal tumors to differentiate unilateral vs. bilateral cortisol hypersecretion.	Catheterization of adrenal veins to measure cortisol and confirm lateralization.	A cortisol adrenal-to-peripheral gradient >6.5 suggests cortisol-secreting adenoma; lateralization ratio ≥ 2.3 indicates unilateral secretion.

CS, Cushing syndrome; CD, Cushing disease (ACTH secreting pituitary adenoma); ULN, Upper limit of normal; DST, Dexamethasone suppression test; HPA axis, Hypothalamic-pituitary-adrenal axis; NET, Neuroendocrine tumor; CBG, Corticosteroid-binding globulin; UFC, Urinary free cortisol; ACTH-dependent CS, Pituitary or ectopic ACTH CS; ACTH-independent CS, Adrenal or exogenous steroid source; BIPSS, Bilateral inferior petrosal sinus sampling.

Table 2.
The main baseline and dynamic hormonal tests used in the diagnosis of Cushing's syndrome.

The *diagnostic approach* involves three key steps: first, excluding exogenous Cushing syndrome; second, confirming the presence of autonomous endogenous cortisol excess; and third, localizing the source of hypercortisolism to guide appropriate therapeutic intervention. In patients with high clinical suspicion for Cushing syndrome but inconclusive or negative test results, repeat testing is recommended in 3 to 6 months, as untreated hypercortisolism can have serious adverse effects [33].

The most common cause of Cushing syndrome is *iatrogenic*, resulting from exogenous corticosteroid use *via* any route (inhaled, topical, parenteral, intra-articular). Identifying exogenous Cushing syndrome through medical history is essential before further diagnostic testing. These patients typically have suppressed serum ACTH, and cortisol levels may be high (due to hydrocortisone use or assay cross-reactivity) or low.

Pseudo-Cushing syndrome, or physiological/non-neoplastic hypercortisolism, occurs in conditions with reactive HPA axis activation, such as pregnancy, alcohol use disorder, obesity, insulin resistance, poorly controlled diabetes, sleep apnea, neuropsychiatric disorders (especially major depression), physical stress, malnutrition, intense exercise, or hypothalamic amenorrhea. Unlike true Cushing syndrome, these patients rarely exhibit characteristic skin or muscle findings [34]. In ambiguous cases, midnight serum cortisol, late-night salivary cortisol, CRH after dexamethasone, or desmopressin testing can help distinguish pseudo-Cushing from true Cushing syndrome [35].

3.2 Hormonal assessment

Urinary-free cortisol. Urinary cortisol excretion over 24 hours is a practical and reliable indicator of serum-free cortisol levels and secretion. Collection instructions: For a 24-hour urine collection, the patient discards the first morning void (noting the time), then collects all urine for the next 24 hours, including urine passed with bowel movements. The collection ends with the first void the following morning, ideally within 10 minutes of the start time. Proper patient instruction is essential, and 24-hour urinary creatinine should be measured to verify specimen completeness. Interpretation: Screening for Cushing syndrome is positive if two urinary cortisol samples are more than three times the upper limit of normal (ULN), or if one sample is ≥ULN and another test is abnormal. Equivocal results (above normal but less than three times ULN) may reflect physiologic hypercortisolism; such cases warrant retesting after several weeks or further diagnostic evaluation [36].

Late night salivary/serum cortisol. Measurement of late-evening salivary or serum cortisol relies on the normal circadian nadir in cortisol, which is preserved in physiologic hypercortisolism but absent in Cushing syndrome. This test is not reliable for patients with irregular sleep schedules or shift work.

Late-night salivary cortisol: Collected at home between 11 PM and midnight using a provided kit. Patients abstain from eating, drinking, smoking, or brushing their teeth for 30 minutes prior to sampling and begin by washing their hands. Following the kit-specific instructions, the provided swab is placed in the mouth to allow passive saturation with saliva, taking care to avoid hand contact. Once adequately saturated, the swab is returned to the collection tube, sealed securely, labeled with the exact collection time, and stored under refrigeration until delivery to the laboratory. Interpretation requires assay- and age-specific reference values due to variability among assays.

Late-night serum cortisol: Typically performed in a hospital setting, often with IV cannula placement to reduce stress artifacts. A bedtime serum cortisol >7.5 mcg/dL (207 nmol/L) suggests Cushing syndrome [36].

Both 24-hour urinary-free cortisol (UFC) and late-night cortisol measurements should be performed at least twice, as cortisol secretion can be variable in Cushing syndrome. Two abnormal results are required to confirm hypercortisolism.

Dexamethasone suppression tests. Dexamethasone is a potent synthetic corticosteroid with minimal mineralocorticoid activity that does not interfere with cortisol measurement in plasma, urine, or saliva. The dexamethasone suppression test diagnoses endogenous Cushing syndrome by evaluating the failure of the HPA axis to suppress cortisol in response to exogenous corticosteroids [37]. Dexamethasone bioavailability may be altered by malabsorption, metabolic changes, or non-compliance. CYP3A4 inducers (e.g., phenytoin, carbamazepine) and inhibitors (e.g., itraconazole, fluoxetine, ritonavir) can affect dexamethasone clearance, risking false results. Measuring serum dexamethasone alongside cortisol helps address this issue [38]. Several dexamethasone suppression test protocols are commonly used in clinical practice.

Low-dose dexamethasone suppression test: serves as screening or diagnostic tool for Cushing syndrome and may be conducted using either an overnight or a two-day protocol.

- Overnight 1 mg test: a single oral dose of 1 mg dexamethasone is administered between 11 PM and midnight, with serum cortisol levels assessed at 8–9 AM the next day.

- Two-day 2 mg test: Dexamethasone 0.5 mg is given orally every 6 hours over a 48-hour period (typically at 9 AM, 3 PM, 9 PM, and 3 AM, total 4 mg); serum cortisol is measured 6 hours after the last dose, usually at 9 AM.

Interpretation: Serum cortisol <1.8 mcg/dL indicates adequate suppression of the hypothalamic-pituitary-adrenal axis and excludes Cushing syndrome [32].

ACTH and DHEA-S. After confirming Cushing syndrome, plasma ACTH is measured to distinguish ACTH-independent (low/undetectable ACTH, adrenal origin) from ACTH-dependent (normal/high ACTH, pituitary, or ectopic origin) cases. Persistently low serum ACTH levels (<5 pg./mL) strongly indicate ACTH-independent CS, most commonly caused by adrenal cortisol-producing lesions, including adrenal adenoma, adrenal carcinoma, or bilateral adrenal hyperplasia, although exogenous glucocorticoid exposure should also be considered. Consistently elevated ACTH (>20 pg./mL) is highly suggestive of ACTH-dependent hypercortisolism, which is typically due to pituitary corticotroph adenomas (Cushing disease) or ectopic ACTH secretion from neuroendocrine tumors, such as small-cell lung carcinoma or bronchial carcinoids (paraneoplastic Cushing syndrome). For intermediate ACTH values (5–20 pg./mL), further dynamic testing—such as CRH, vasopressin (desmopressin) stimulation tests—is required. In these tests, a significant rise in ACTH and cortisol following stimulation supports a pituitary source (Cushing disease), whereas a blunted or absent response favors adrenal causes or most ectopic ACTH-producing tumors (further details regarding the methodology and interpretation of the desmopressin stimulation test are provided below). Repeated measurement of serum DHEA-S may also help; levels are typically suppressed in ACTH-independent Cushing syndrome because of chronic ACTH inhibition, while they are normal or elevated in ACTH-dependent forms, reflecting the sustained ACTH stimulation [39].

High-dose dexamethasone suppression test (HDDST). In ACTH-dependent Cushing syndrome, the HDDST helps differentiate pituitary (Cushing disease) from ectopic ACTH production. Only pituitary ACTH secretion is typically partially or fully suppressed by high-dose dexamethasone (8 mg).

- Overnight 8 mg test: Baseline morning cortisol is measured; 8 mg oral dexamethasone is taken at 11 PM–midnight, and cortisol is measured between 8 and 9 AM the next morning.

- Two-day 8 mg test: On day 1, baseline morning serum cortisol or 24-hour urinary-free cortisol from the previous day is obtained. Dexamethasone 2 mg is given orally every 6 hours for 2 days (total 16 mg); urinary-free cortisol is collected on the second day or serum cortisol is measured after the final dexamethasone dose.

Interpretation: A > 50% reduction in urinary-free or serum cortisol suggests a pituitary source (Cushing disease) [12]. However, lack of suppression does not exclude Cushing disease, as some pituitary tumors are resistant to dexamethasone.

Dexamethasone-suppressed corticotropin-releasing hormone (CRH) test. This combined test is considered the most effective dynamic test for distinguishing Cushing disease from physiologic hypercortisolism (pseudo-Cushing syndrome). The protocol involves administering dexamethasone 0.5 mg orally every 6 hours for 48 hours, then administering 1 mcg/kg IV CRH 2 hours after the final dexamethasone dose, typically at 8 AM. Serum cortisol is measured 15 minutes after CRH administration. Interpretation: A serum cortisol >1.4 mcg/dL (39 nmol/L) 15 minutes later supports a diagnosis of Cushing disease [40].

Desmopressin test. Desmopressin, a synthetic analog of arginine-vasopressin, can stimulate ACTH secretion from pituitary tumors expressing aberrant V3 receptors. The test involves collecting baseline ACTH and cortisol, then administering 10 μg IV desmopressin in the morning after an overnight fast, with additional samples at 15-, 30-, 45-, 60-, 90-, and 120-minute post-injection. A 20% rise in serum cortisol and 50% increase in plasma ACTH suggest Cushing disease. However, some ectopic tumors may also respond, so interpretation should be in conjunction with other tests, such as the HDDST [41]. Combined criteria (20% cortisol and 30% ACTH rise with 50% cortisol suppression on HDDST) provide high specificity for Cushing disease [42].

Bilateral inferior petrosal sinus sampling (BIPSS) is the gold standard for distinguishing Cushing disease from ectopic ACTH-dependent Cushing syndrome by assessing the central-to-peripheral ACTH gradient. The procedure is typically performed with CRH stimulation; a central-to-peripheral (C:P) ACTH ratio > 2 at baseline or > 3 after CRH suggests a pituitary source, and an interpetrosal ratio ≥ 1.4 aids in lateralization [36]. Due to limited CRH availability and varying sensitivity, desmopressin (DDAVP) is increasingly used as an alternative stimulant. With desmopressin, ACTH samples are collected from bilateral petrosal sinuses and a peripheral vein at baseline and at 3-, 5-, and 10-minute post-injection of 10 μg IV desmopressin. A recent study reports that optimal C:P ratio cutoffs are 1.4 before and 2.8 after stimulation [43]. False negatives may occur due to anatomical or biochemical disease variations.

Adrenal vein sampling (AVS) is indicated for patients with ACTH-independent Cushing's syndrome who present with bilateral adrenal tumors on imaging, where the differential diagnosis includes unilateral or bilateral cortisol-secreting adenomas, macronodular adrenal hyperplasia, or primary pigmented nodular adrenocortical disease. AVS helps distinguish among these conditions by directly measuring cortisol secretion from each adrenal gland. The procedure is performed by an interventional radiologist under sedation, typically in the morning following an overnight fast and after administration of dexamethasone to suppress endogenous ACTH. The adrenal veins are catheterized *via* the femoral vein, with correct catheter placement confirmed by venogram. Blood samples are collected from both adrenal veins and the external iliac vein, and analyzed for cortisol and aldosterone levels. Complications are rare but can include thrombosis, adrenal insufficiency, or hypertensive crisis. Notably, aldosterone levels tend to be higher in the right adrenal vein due to anatomical differences, limiting its use for correcting dilution between sides; plasma epinephrine is used to confirm catheterization success instead. A successful AVS is indicated by adrenal vein aldosterone concentrations exceeding peripheral levels by over 100 pg./ml. A cortisol gradient (adrenal-to-peripheral) over 6.5 suggests a cortisol-secreting adenoma. Lateralization is determined by a side-to-side cortisol ratio of 2.3 or higher, indicating predominant secretion from one adrenal gland [44].

3.3 Evaluation of hypercortisolism in special populations

- Abnormal CBG: Late-night salivary cortisol or urinary-free cortisol (UFC) is preferred. Estrogen therapy should be discontinued at least 6 weeks before dexamethasone suppression testing (DST).

- Cyclic Cushing syndrome: Characterized by intermittent episodes of cortisol excess. UFC or late-night salivary cortisol is preferred for diagnosis, with repeat testing if initial results are normal but suspicion remains high. True cyclic CS is rare, but cortisol variability is frequent in all CS etiologies.

- In patients with chronic kidney disease, use the 1 mg overnight DST instead of UFC.

- For patients with epilepsy, UFC or bedtime salivary cortisol is preferred over DST, as antiseizure medications increase dexamethasone clearance.

3.4 Imaging studies in ACTH-dependent Cushing syndrome

- Cross-sectional imaging: Magnetic resonance imaging (MRI) is the preferred method for localizing ACTH-producing pituitary adenomas [45]. Tumors >10 mm are considered the source of ACTH, warranting pituitary surgery. For smaller lesions, further diagnostics are needed to differentiate pituitary from ectopic ACTH sources. Whole-body CT scans are used to localize ectopic ACTH-secreting tumors.

- Functional imaging: 11C-methionine PET (Met-PET) can detect small ACTH-producing pituitary tumors. When ectopic ACTH syndrome is suspected but cross-sectional imaging is negative, somatostatin analog scintigraphy (68Ga-DOTA-somatostatin analog PET/CT or 111In-pentetreotide SPECT/CT) offers high sensitivity (88–93%). 18F-FDG PET/CT is primarily used for grade 3 neuroendocrine tumors or carcinomas [45].

4. Conclusions

Dynamic testing is central to the accurate diagnosis and differential assessment of both adrenal insufficiency and Cushing syndrome, especially when basal hormone measurements yield inconclusive results. In adrenal insufficiency, dynamic stimulation tests—such as the standard high-dose ACTH stimulation test, insulin tolerance test, and metyrapone test—are essential for confirming deficient adrenal reserve and distinguishing between primary and secondary causes. Each test has distinct indications, limitations, and interpretation criteria, emphasizing the need for careful patient selection and consideration of confounding factors. In the evaluation of Cushing syndrome, dynamic suppression, and stimulation protocols, including dexamethasone suppression tests, CRH and desmopressin stimulation, bilateral inferior petrosal sinus sampling and adrenal venous sampling, are critical for confirming endogenous hypercortisolism, differentiating ACTH-dependent from ACTH-independent etiologies, and localizing the source of excess hormone production. The integration of dynamic testing results with clinical findings and imaging studies ensures precise diagnosis, guiding targeted management and improving patient outcomes. Ultimately, understanding the principles, protocols, and pitfalls of dynamic testing is essential for all clinicians and laboratory specialists involved in the assessment of HPA axis disorders.

Conflict of interest

The authors declare no conflicts of interest.
Both authors contributed equally to the preparation of this chapter.

Author details

Daniela Greere and Diana Loreta Păun*
Carol Davila University of Medicine and Pharmacy, The University Emergency Hospital, Bucharest, Romania

*Address all correspondence to: dianaloreta_paun@yahoo.com

References

[1] Melmed S, Koenig R, Rosen C, Auchus R, Goldfine A. Williams Textbook of Endocrinology. 14th ed. Philadelphia, PA: Elsevier; 2020

[2] Bansal V, Asmar NE, Selman WR, Arafah BM. Pitfalls in the diagnosis and management of Cushing's syndrome. Neurosurgical Focus. 2015;**38**(2):E4. DOI: 10.3171/2014.11.focus14704

[3] Bornstein SR, Allolio B, Arlt W, Barthel A, Don-Wauchope A, Hammer GD, et al. Diagnosis and treatment of primary adrenal insufficiency: An endocrine society clinical practice guideline. The Journal of Clinical Endocrinology & Metabolism. 2016;**101**(2):364-389. DOI: 10.1210/jc.2015-1710

[4] Beuschlein F, Else T, Bancos I, Hahner S, Hamidi O, van Hulsteijn L, et al. European Society of Endocrinology and Endocrine Society Joint Clinical Guideline: Diagnosis and therapy of glucocorticoid-induced adrenal insufficiency. European Journal of Endocrinology. 2024;**190**(5):G25-G51. DOI: 10.1093/ejendo/lvae029

[5] Speiser PW, Arlt W, Auchus RJ, Baskin LS, Conway GS, Merke DP, et al. Congenital adrenal hyperplasia due to steroid 21-hydroxylase deficiency: An Endocrine Society* Clinical Practice Guideline. The Journal of Clinical Endocrinology & Metabolism. 2018;**103**(11):4043-4088. DOI: 10.1210/jc.2018-01865

[6] Mathara Diddhenipothage SAD, Beck KJ, Loo H, Amiyangoda GK, Pofi R, Tomlinson JW, et al. "A morning cortisol is the most effective clinical predictor of short synacthen test outcome": A tertiary care centre experience. Clinical Endocrinology. 2023;**99**(2):142-151. DOI: 10.1111/cen.14934

[7] Schmidt IL, Lahner H, Mann K, Petersenn S. Diagnosis of adrenal insufficiency: Evaluation of the corticotropin-releasing hormone test and basal serum cortisol in comparison to the insulin tolerance test in patients with hypothalamic-pituitary-adrenal disease. The Journal of Clinical Endocrinology & Metabolism. 2003;**88**(9):4193-4198. DOI: 10.1210/jc.2002-021897

[8] Uslar T, Olmos R, Martínez-Aguayo A, Baudrand R. Clinical update on congenital adrenal hyperplasia: Recommendations from a multidisciplinary adrenal program. Journal of Clinical Medicine. 2023;**12**(9):3128. DOI: 10.3390/jcm12093128

[9] Yau M, Gujral J, New MI. In: Feingold KR, Anawalt B, Boyce A, Chrousos G, de Herder WW, Dungan K, et al., editors. Congenital Adrenal Hyperplasia: Diagnosis and Emergency Treatment. [Internet]. South Dartmouth (MA): MDText.com, Inc.; 2019. Available from: https:ncbi.nlm.nih.gov/books/NBK279085/

[10] Al-Aridi R, Abdelmannan D, Arafah B. Biochemical diagnosis of adrenal insufficiency: The added value of dehydroepiandrosterone sulfate measurements. Endocrine Practice. 2011;**17**(2):261-270. DOI: 10.4158/ep10262.ra

[11] Han AJ, Suresh M, Gruber L, Algeciras-Schimnich A, Achenbach SJ, Atkinson EJ, et al. Performance of dehydroepiandrosterone sulfate and baseline cortisol in assessing adrenal

insufficiency. The Journal of Clinical Endocrinology & Metabolism. 2025;**110**(9):e3117-e3124. DOI: 10.1210/clinem/dgae855

[12] Yeo JKT, Babic N, Hannoush ZC, Weiss RE. In: Feingold KR, Anawalt B, Boyce A, Chrousos G, Dungan K, Grossman A, et al., editors. Endocrine Testing Protocols: Hypothalamic Pituitary Adrenal Axis [Internet]. South Dartmouth (MA): MDText.com, Inc.; 2000. Available from: https://www.ncbi.nlm.nih.gov/books/NBK278940/

[13] Javorsky BR, Raff H, Carroll TB, Algeciras-Schimnich A, Singh RJ, Colón-Franco JM, et al. New Cutoffs for the biochemical diagnosis of adrenal insufficiency after ACTH stimulation using specific cortisol assays. Journal of the Endocrine Society. 2021;**5**(4):bvab022. DOI: 10.1210/jendso/bvab022

[14] Qureshi AC, Bahri A, Breen LA, Barnes SC, Powrie JK, Thomas SM, et al. The influence of the route of oestrogen administration on serum levels of cortisol-binding globulin and total cortisol. Clinical Endocrinology. 2007;**66**(5):632-635. DOI: 10.1111/j.1365-2265.2007.02784.x

[15] Ergin AB, Kennedy AL, Gupta MK, Hamrahian AH. The Cleveland Clinic Manual of Dynamic Endocrine Testing. Cham: Springer International Publishing; 2015

[16] Stathori G, Alexakis D, Chrousos GP, Paltoglou G. Examining aldosterone plasma concentration alterations post-ACTH stimulation in healthy subjects: A systematic literature review and meta-analysis on ACTH's role in aldosterone secretion. Hormones (Athens). 2024;**23**(4):765-775. DOI: 10.1007/s42000-024-00583-6

[17] Sobolewska J, Dzialach L, Kuca P, Witek P. Critical illness-related corticosteroid insufficiency - An overview of pathogenesis, clinical presentation and management. Frontiers in Endocrinology. 2024;**15**:1473151. DOI: 10.3389/fendo.2024.1473151

[18] Dökmetaş HS, Çolak R, Keleştimur F, Selçuklu A, Ünlühizarci K, Bayram F. A comparison between the 1-µg adrenocorticotropin (ACTH) test, the short ACTH (250 µg) test, and the insulin tolerance test in the assessment of hypothalamo-pituitary-adrenal axis immediately after pituitary surgery. The Journal of Clinical Endocrinology & Metabolism. 2000;**85**(10):3713-3719. DOI: 10.1210/jcem.85.10.6879

[19] Erturk E, Jaffe CA, Barkan AL. Evaluation of the integrity of the hypothalamic-pituitary-adrenal axis by insulin hypoglycemia test. The Journal of Clinical Endocrinology & Metabolism. 1998;**83**(7):2350-2354. DOI: 10.1210/jcem.83.7.4980

[20] Staub JJ, Jenkins JS, Ratcliffe JG, Landon J. Comparison of corticotrophin and corticosteroid response to lysine vasopressin, insulin, and pyrogen in man. BMJ British Medical Journal. 1973;**1**(5848):267-269. DOI: 10.1136/bmj.1.5848.267

[21] Karpman MS, Neculau M, Dias VC, Kline GA. Defining adrenal status with salivary cortisol by gold-standard insulin hypoglycemia. Clinical Biochemistry. 2013;**46**(15):1442-1446. DOI: 10.1016/j.clinbiochem.2013.05.004

[22] Steiner H, Bähr V, Exner P, Oelkers P. Pituitary function tests: Comparison of ACTH and 11-deoxy-cortisol responses in the metyrapone test and with the insulin hypoglycemia test. Experimental and Clinical Endocrinology & Diabetes. 2009;**102**(01):33-38. DOI: 10.1055/s-0029-1211262

[23] Gasco V, Ferrero A, Bisceglia A, Prencipe N, Cambria V, Bioletto F, et al. The cut-off limits of growth hormone response to the insulin tolerance test related to body mass index for the diagnosis of adult growth hormone deficiency. Neuroendocrinology. 2021;**111**(5):442-450. DOI: 10.1159/000508103

[24] Yuen KCJ, Biller BMK, Radovick S, Carmichael JD, Jasim S, Pantalone KM, et al. American Association of Clinical Endocrinologists and American College of endocrinology Guidelines for management of growth hormone deficiency in adults and patients transitioning from pediatric to adult care. Endocrine Practice. 2019;**25**(11):1191-1232. DOI: 10.4158/gl-2019-0405

[25] English K, Inder WJ, Weedon Z, Dimeski G, Sorbello J, Russell AW, et al. Prospective evaluation of a week one overnight metyrapone test with subsequent dynamic assessments of hypothalamic-pituitary-adrenal axis function after pituitary surgery. Clinical Endocrinology. 2017;**87**(3):312-312. DOI: 10.1111/cen.13428

[26] Saini J, Garcia RG, Herndon J, Erickson D, Gruber L, Bancos I. Use of overnight metyrapone test in suspected secondary adrenal insufficiency: A retrospective single Centre-study. Clinical Endocrinology. 2023;**100**(3): 203-211. DOI: 10.1111/cen.14989

[27] Jubiz W, Meikle AW, West CD, Tyler FH. Single-dose metyrapone test. Archives of Internal Medicine [Internet]. 1970;**125**(3):472-474. Available from: https://pubmed.ncbi.nlm.nih.gov/4313728/

[28] Spiger M, Jubiz W, Meikle AW, West CD, Tylor FH. Single-dose metyrapone test: Review of a four-year experience. Archives of Internal Medicine [Internet]. 1975;**135**(5):698-700. Available from: https://pubmed.ncbi.nlm.nih.gov/1052666/

[29] Girard J, Baumann JB, Zuppinger K. Assessment of ACTH-adrenal activity and diagnostic value of plasma ACTH. Pediatric Research. 1979;**13**(10):1196-1196. DOI: 10.1203/00006450-197910000-00093

[30] Lindholm J, Juul S, Jørgensen JOL, Astrup J, Bjerre P, Feldt-Rasmussen U, et al. Incidence and late prognosis of Cushing's syndrome: A population-based study. The Journal of Clinical Endocrinology & Metabolism. 2001;**86**(1):117-123. DOI: 10.1210/jcem.86.1.7093

[31] Wagner-Bartak NA, Baiomy A, Habra MA, Mukhi SV, Morani AC, Korivi BR, et al. Cushing syndrome: Diagnostic workup and imaging features, with clinical and pathologic correlation. American Journal of Roentgenology. 2017;**209**(1):19-32. DOI: 10.2214/ajr.16.17290

[32] Nieman LK, Biller BMK, Findling JW, Newell-Price J, Savage MO, Stewart PM, et al. The diagnosis of Cushing's syndrome: An Endocrine Society Clinical Practice Guideline. The Journal of Clinical Endocrinology & Metabolism. 2008;**93**(5):1526-1540. DOI: 10.1210/jc.2008-0125

[33] Nieman LK. Diagnosis of Cushing's syndrome in the modern era. Endocrinology and Metabolism Clinics of North America. 2018;**47**(2):259-273. DOI: 10.1016/j.ecl.2018.02.001

[34] Chabre O. The difficulties of pseudo-Cushing's syndrome (or "non-neoplastic hypercortisolism"). Annales d'Endocrinologie. 2018;**79**(3):138-145. DOI: 10.1016/j.ando.2018.04.017

[35] Alwani RA, Schmit Jongbloed LW, de Jong FH, van der Lely AJ, de Herder WW, Feelders RA. Differentiating between Cushing's disease and pseudo-Cushing's syndrome: Comparison of four tests. European Journal of Endocrinology. 2014;**170**(4):477-486. DOI: 10.1530/EJE-13-0702

[36] Juszczak A, Sulentic P, Grossman A. In: Feingold KR, Anawalt B, Boyce A, Chrousos G, de Herder WW, Dungan K, et al., editors. Cushing's Syndrome [Internet]. South Dartmouth (MA): MDText.com, Inc.; 2024. Available from: https://www.ncbi.nlm.nih.gov/books/NBK279088/

[37] Keevil BG. Improving the dexamethasone suppression test. Clinical Chemistry. 2021;**67**(7):929-931. DOI: 10.1093/clinchem/hvab076

[38] Aw M. Dexamethasone suppression tests: Usefulness of simultaneous measurement of plasma cortisol and dexamethasone. Clinical Endocrinology. 1982;**16**(4):401-408. DOI: 10.1111/j.1365-2265.1982.tb00733.x

[39] Hong AR, Kim JH, Hong ES, Kim IK, Park KS, Ahn CH, et al. Limited diagnostic utility of plasma adrenocorticotropic hormone for differentiation between adrenal Cushing syndrome and Cushing disease. Endocrinology and Metabolism. 2015;**30**(3):297. DOI: 10.3803/enm.2015.30.3.297

[40] Yanovski JA, Cutler GB, Chrousos GP, Nieman LK. Corticotropin-releasing hormone stimulation following low-dose dexamethasone administration. A new test to distinguish Cushing's syndrome from pseudo-Cushing's states. Journal of the American Medical Association. 1993;**269**(17):2237-2241. DOI: 10.1001/jama.1993.03500170062035

[41] Ceccato F, Barbot M, Mondin A, Boscaro M, Fleseriu M, Scaroni C. Dynamic testing for differential diagnosis of ACTH-dependent Cushing syndrome: A systematic review and meta-analysis. The Journal of Clinical Endocrinology & Metabolism. 2023;**108**(5):e178-e188. DOI: 10.1210/clinem/dgac686

[42] Qiao J, Li J, Zhang W, Wang C, Li J, Jiang S, et al. The usefulness of the combined high-dose dexamethasone suppression test and desmopressin stimulation test in establishing the source of ACTH secretion in ACTH-dependent Cushing's syndrome. Endocrine Journal. 2021;**68**(7):839-848. DOI: 10.1507/endocrj.ej20-0837

[43] Chen S, Chen K, Wang S, Zhu H, Lu L, Zhang X, et al. The optimal cut-off of BIPSS in differential diagnosis of ACTH-dependent Cushing's syndrome: Is stimulation necessary? The Journal of Clinical Endocrinology & Metabolism. 2020;**105**(4):e1673-e1685. DOI: 10.1210/clinem/dgz194

[44] Wiggam MI, Heaney AP, McIlrath EM, McCance DR, Sheridan B, Hadden DR, et al. Bilateral inferior petrosal sinus sampling in the differential diagnosis of adrenocorticotropin-dependent Cushing's syndrome: A comparison with other diagnostic tests. The Journal of Clinical Endocrinology & Metabolism. 2000;**85**(4):1525-1532. DOI: 10.1210/jcem.85.4.6574

[45] Senanayake R, Gillett D, MacFarlane J, Van de Meulen M, Powlson A, Koulouri O, et al. New types of localization methods for adrenocorticotropic hormone-dependent Cushing's syndrome. Best Practice & Research Clinical Endocrinology & Metabolism. 2021;**35**(1):101513. DOI: 10.1016/j.beem.2021.101513

Chapter 5

Adrenal Insufficiency Associated with Inhaled Corticosteroid Use

Esha Elizabeth Cherian and Jubbin Jagan Jacob

Abstract

Inhaled corticosteroids (ICS) are the first-line treatment for persistent asthma and chronic respiratory diseases due to their strong local anti-inflammatory effects and better safety profile compared to systemic corticosteroids. However, their use for a long period, especially at higher doses or together with other corticosteroid products, can lead to suppression of the hypothalamic-pituitary-adrenal (HPA) axis and cause secondary adrenal insufficiency. This is not a well-known clinical problem because of its gradual onset and nonspecific symptoms, but it can lead to serious health issues such as adrenal crisis during physiological stress. This chapter encapsulates all aspects of adrenal insufficiency associated with inhaled corticosteroids, starting with HPA axis physiology and ICS pharmacokinetics and pharmacodynamics. The chapter describes the current algorithms for pathophysiology, clinical presentation, the diagnostic approach, and ICS-induced adrenal insufficiency along with management strategies that are based on the latest clinical guidelines. There is strong focus on the risk stratification, recommended regular monitoring, and prevention strategies to minimize HPA axis suppression due to ICS. The clinical applications of these topics are clearly depicted in algorithms, tables, and infographics to maximize the reader's comprehension. Due to the prevalent usage of inhaled corticosteroids in both adults and pediatric population for the management of various obstructive respiratory illnesses, it is crucial to identify and proactively manage adrenal insufficiency to ensure patient safety while not compromising on controlling the disease.

Keywords: inhaled corticosteroids, adrenal insufficiency, HPA axis suppression, asthma, pediatric endocrinology, adrenal crisis, corticosteroid tapering

1. Introduction

Inhaled corticosteroids (ICS) are a widely used treatment option for a number of obstructive airway diseases—the most common of which are Bronchial Asthma (BA) and Chronic Obstructive Pulmonary Disease (COPD). ICS are given to patients through a local route of administration; however, with prolonged use, they do exert major systemic side effects such as suppression of the hypothalamic-pituitary-adrenal (HPA) axis that ultimately can manifest as secondary adrenal insufficiency (AI). It is an iatrogenic complication of ICS that poses a major diagnostic challenge due to its subacute presentation and nonspecific clinical symptoms. In severe cases, it can lead to life-threatening adrenal crises, the risk of the which is heightened in those receiving higher dosages, among pediatric population, or patients that are simultaneously prescribed additional medication that affect corticosteroid metabolism (such as CYP3A4 inhibitors) [1–12].

This chapter highlights the mechanistic pathways of corticosteroid-induced adrenal insufficiency along with its clinical features, diagnosis, and management.

2. Physiology of hypothalamic pituitary adrenal (HPA) axis

The hypothalamic-pituitary axis is a neuroendocrine pathway, the primary function of which is to regulate our body's response to both internal and external stress

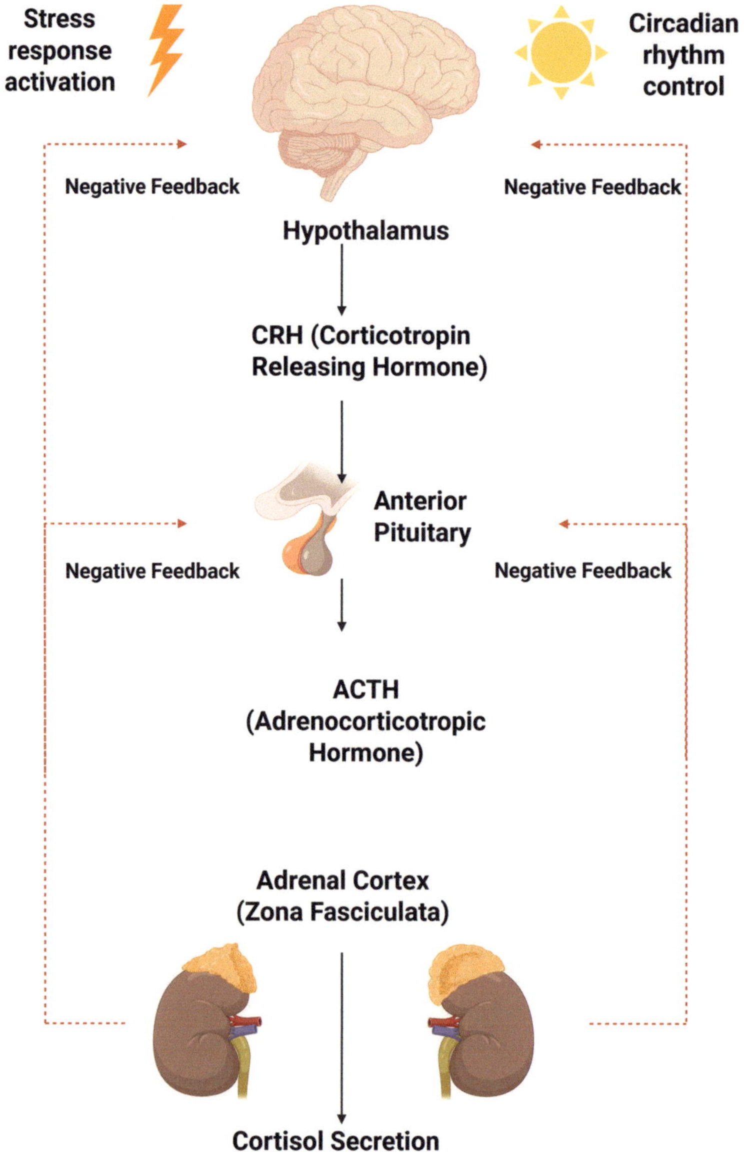

Figure 1.
Physiology of hypothalamic pituitary adrenal axis. Created in BioRender. Cherian [14] https://BioRender.com/qpccrhg.

in order to maintain proper homeostasis. It begins in the hypothalamus that secretes corticotropin-releasing hormone (CRH) in response to our body's natural circadian rhythm and stress factors [13]. This in turn stimulates the anterior part of the pituitary gland in order to release adrenocorticotropic hormone (ACTH). ACTH then proceeds to act on the cortex (the zona fasciculata) of the adrenal gland to synthesize and secrete glucocorticoids—mainly cortisol that plays a vital role in the maintenance of several physiological processes including our body's metabolism, electrolyte imbalance, immune function, as well as cardiovascular tone. Cortisol regulates its own production through a negative feedback mechanism exerted upon both the hypothalamus and pituitary gland to prevent excessive hormone release [2]. Cortisol release is dependent upon the body's natural circadian rhythm. Cortisol secretion spikes in the early mornings, reaching its peak around 6–8 AM, and then plateaus around midnight (**Figure 1**) [2–4].

However, in stressful situations, the body releases ultradian pulses that stimulate the release of excess ACTH and cortisol to manage the body's heightened physiological demands. The mechanism for the development of secondary adrenal insufficiency in patients with asthma or COPD is brought about when they take high dosages of exogenous corticosteroids for prolonged periods of time that suppresses the HPA axis by imitating cortisol's feedback mechanism. This suppression leads to decreased endogenous corticosteroid production by reducing the stimulation of the adrenal cortex by ACTH and, ultimately, adrenal atrophy [2, 3].

3. Pharmacokinetics and pharmacodynamics of inhaled corticosteroids

Inhaled corticosteroids are designed to provide powerful anti-inflammatory effects to the airways with the least possible exposure to the rest of the body. However, some corticosteroids will reach the body's systemic circulation, making pharmacokinetic and pharmacodynamic understanding necessary to appreciate the effects on the hypothalamic-pituitary-adrenal (HPA) axis suppression risk (**Figure 2**) [5, 6, 9, 12].

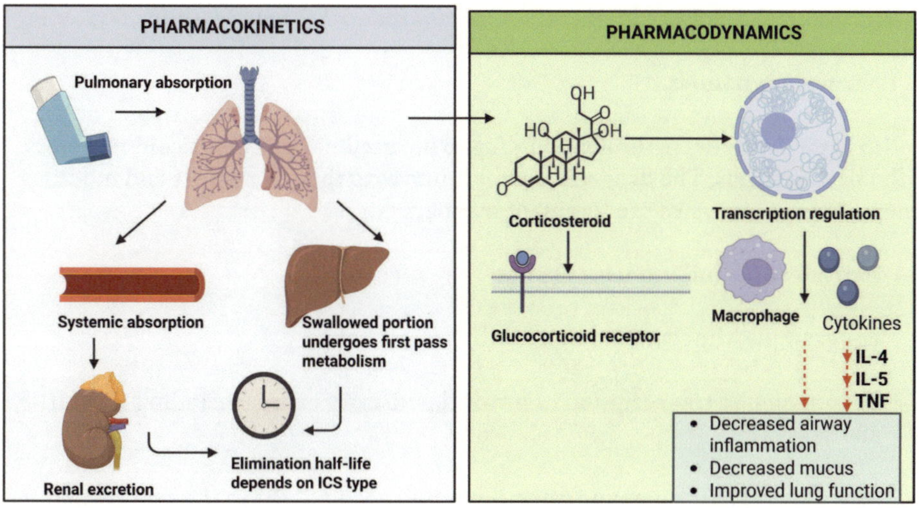

Figure 2.
Pharmacokinetics and pharmacodynamics of ICS. Created in BioRender. Cherian [15] https://BioRender.com/oowov2g.

3.1 Pharmacokinetics

3.1.1 Absorption

Inhaled corticosteroids (ICS) are administered through metered dose inhalers (MDIs), dry powder inhalers (DPIs), or nebulizers. After inhalation, drug particles settle in the bronchial tree and are absorbed into the pulmonary circulation. A considerable portion, especially with poor inhaler technique, settles in the oropharynx, is swallowed, and enters the gastrointestinal tract. The pulmonary portion bypasses the first-pass metabolism, and the absorbed drug is rapidly distributed to the circulation. The swallowed portion is first metabolized in the liver before reaching circulation.

3.1.2 Distribution

ICS, like other inhaled corticosteroids, are bound to plasma proteins (up to 90%); inhaled corticosteroids have very high protein binding. Lipophilic compounds (fluticasone, mometasone) are more readily absorbed to the airway tissues and retained longer, increasing local and systemic exposure [5, 6, 9, 10, 16, 17].

3.1.3 Metabolism

Most inhaled corticosteroids (ICS) are metabolized through the liver's cytochrome P450 3A4 (CYP3A4) enzyme system. Strong CYP3A4 enzyme inhibitors like ritonavir and ketoconazole may substantially elevate systemic steroid concentrations, thus increasing the likelihood of HPA axis suppression [2, 3, 5, 6, 9, 10].

3.1.4 Elimination

After hepatic metabolism, ICS are primarily eliminated through the biliary system, with only minute amounts excreted renally. The plasma half-life shows variability among different agents; for instance, fluticasone propionate has a systemic half-life of approximately 7–8 hours while budesonide's is around 2–3 hours [10, 16, 17].

3.2 Pharmacodynamics

ICS exert their effects through binding to intracellular glucocorticoid receptors (GRs) of target cells. The drug-GR complex moves to the cell nucleus and modifies gene transcription in two predominant manners:

1. Activates anti-inflammatory genes

   For example,- lipocortin-1 that inhibits phospholipase A2.

2. Suppression of transcription of pro-inflammatory genes (including IL-4, IL-5, and TNF-α).

These changes in the genome cause decreased eosinophilia in the airways and edema of the mucosa and better airway hyperresponsiveness.

Non-genomic effects, including vasoconstriction of airway microvasculature, may manifest within minutes.

3.2.1 HPA Axis blockage

Long-term exposure, especially to high dosages or strong compounds, can cause systemic absorption that is strong enough to shut down the hypothalamic–pituitary–adrenal (HPA) axis, which lowers the body's natural production of cortisol. Children, the elderly, and people who are already taking CYP3A4 inhibitors are at a higher risk.

4. Pathophysiology of ICS induced adrenal insufficiency

The hypothalamic–pituitary–adrenal (HPA) axis manages cortisol secretion under normal physiological conditions through a feedback control mechanism [2, 3].

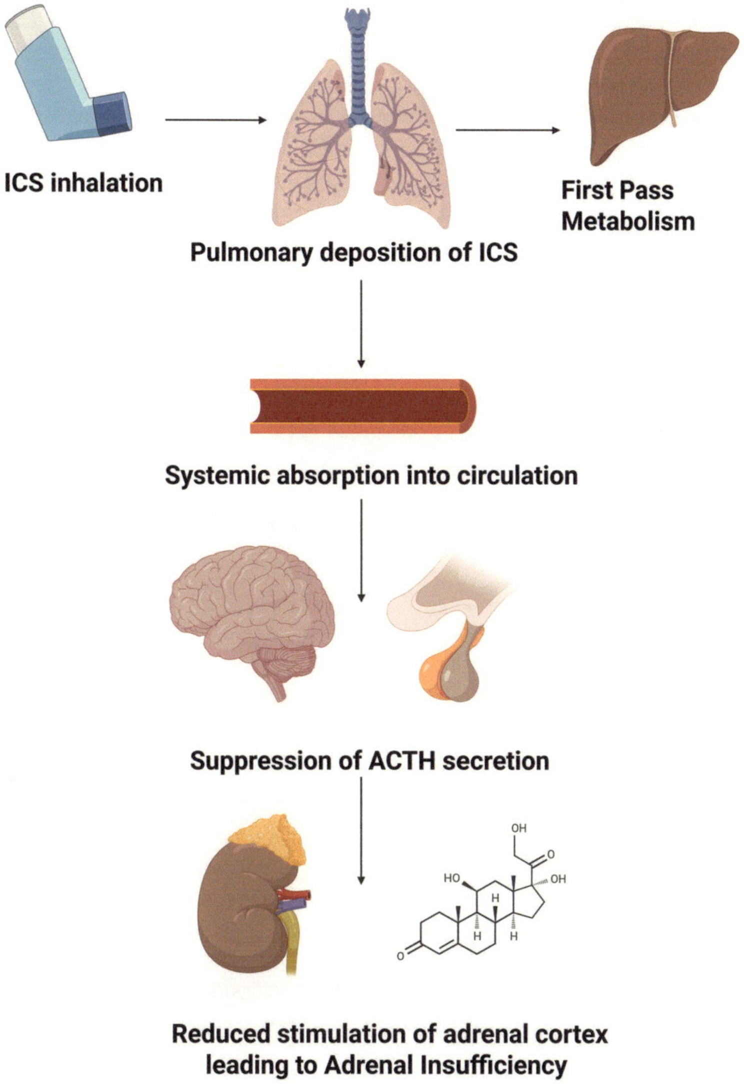

Figure 3.
Pathophysiology of ICS induced Adrenal Insufficiency. Created in BioRender. Cherian [19, 20] https://BioRender.com/rft2wev.

The hypothalamus releases Corticotropin-releasing hormone (CRH) following the body's natural circadian rhythms as well as during physiological stress and in turn prompts the anterior pituitary to release adrenocorticotropic hormone (ACTH). Subsequently, cortisol is produced by the adrenal cortex (specifically zona fasciculata) in response to ACTH. Circulating cortisol inhibits the release of both hypothalamic CRH and pituitary ACTH through a negative feedback loop, thereby restoring the balance of the hormones present.

ICS have a primary use as anti-inflammatory agents for the local treatment of inflammation in the lungs. However, as is the case with ICS, a significant portion of the prescribed dose is often swallowed and subsequently absorbed through the gastrointestinal tract, alongside some being absorbed systemically through the pulmonary vasculature. This becomes clinically significant when ICS, particularly fluticasone and ciclesonide [18], are prescribed. Both of these drugs are potent ICS with strong glucocorticoid receptor affinity, long half-lives, and are resistant to hepatic first-pass metabolism. The combination of these properties increases systemic bioavailability and the risk of HPA axis suppression, more so with increased ICS dose or with longer treatment duration (**Figure 3**) [2–6, 9, 10, 12, 16, 17].

Circulating exogenous corticosteroids act as feedback for the endogenous cortisol pathways. They inhibit the release of CRH from the hypothalamus as well as ACTH from the anterior pituitary. Eventually, this leads to the peripherally acting corticosteroids administering diminished stimulation to the adrenal cortex resulting in cortical atrophy and suppressed cortisol production. This form of suppression remains clinically silent until exposed to a physiological stressor such as infection, trauma, or surgery; then, the inability of the adrenals to respond to stress with adequate cortisol may lead to adrenal crisis. Notably, mineralocorticoid secretion can escape ICS induced adrenal insufficiency and remains normal as ICS suppression occurs due to the primary regulation from the renin–angiotensin–aldosterone system (RAAS), differing from primary adrenal insufficiency. HPA axis recovery post ICS tapering remains unpredictable [1–3, 7, 8].

5. Clinical presentation of adrenal insufficiency

5.1 Clinical features

5.1.1 Symptoms

- Chronic fatigue
- Weight loss and decreased appetite
- Gastrointestinal symptoms- > nausea, abdominal pain, vomiting, diarrhea, or constipation
- Postural hypotension or dizziness
- Neuropsychiatric disturbances: irritability, depression, or apathy
- Myalgia
- Arthralgia
- Lethargy

5.1.2 Signs

- Hyponatremia
- Hyperkalemia (rare)
- Hypoglycemia
- CBC and DLC - > Eosinophilia, lymphocytosis, and anemia
- Mild hypercalcemia
- Thyroid function tests - > mildly elevated TSH

The differences between primary and secondary adrenal insufficiency are tabulated in **Table 1**.

5.1.3 Clinical features in pediatrics

The clinical presentation may be subtle and tends to be nonspecific in nature [7, 11, 21];

- Increased tiredness, weakness, fatigue, decreased appetite.
- Deceleration in growth or delayed in the onset of puberty.
- Head and abdominal pain.
- Low blood sugar, especially during changes in health status.
- Episodes of nonspecific vomiting.

Clinical features	Primary AI (Adrenal gland failure)	Secondary AI (HPA Axis suppression)
Pathology	Damage to adrenal cortex	Reduced ACTH secretion from pituitary (or CRH from hypothalamus)
Onset	Gradual (may be acute in crisis)	Gradual (often unmasked during stress)
Skin changes	Hyperpigmentation (Increased ACTH & MSH)	Usually absent (low ACTH)
Electrolyte changes	Hyponatremia, hyperkalemia (loss of aldosterone)	Hyponatremia possible Potassium is usually normal
Hypoglycemia	Common	Common (especially in children)
Blood pressure	Often low (may worsen in crisis)	Low (milder hypotension)
Cortisol levels	Low	Low
ACTH levels	High	Low or inappropriately normal)
Aldosterone levels	Low	Normal
Response to ACTH stimulation test	Blunted or absent	Often blunted but may be partial if suppression is incomplete

Table 1.
Comparison between primary and secondary adrenal insufficiency.

5.2 Adrenal crisis

Adrenal crisis (acute adrenal insufficiency) is an acute, severe, and life-threatening deficiency of cortisol levels within the body. In relation to the use of inhaled corticosteroids, this condition may develop when there is inadequate stress response to illness, surgery, trauma, or steroid withdrawal due to HPA axis suppression [2, 3, 5–9].

5.2.1 Precipitating factors

- Severe infection like gastroenteritis or pneumonia
- Surgery or major trauma
- Cessation or tapering corticosteroids too fast
- Sustained vomiting or diarrhea that prevents oral steroid consumption

5.2.2 Primary symptoms

- Severe and persistent fatigue
- Nausea and vomiting
- Abdominal pain

5.2.3 Intermediate symptoms

- Hypotension (in some cases may progress to shock)
- Severe dehydration
- Altered mental status - > including confusion, delirium, staggered consciousness, or even coma
- Fever (in the presence of infection)

5.2.4 Laboratory findings

- Hyponatremia
- Low blood glucose
- Increased levels of creatinine and urea (due to dehydration).

5.2.5 Management

- IV Hydrocortisone 100 mg bolus then continuous or IV every 6–8 hrs. [1, 7]
- IV isotonic saline for hypervolemia.

- Sepsis should be treated with appropriate antibiotic
- Hypoglycemia should be corrected

6. Diagnosis of ICS associated adrenal insufficiency

Diagnosing ICS associated adrenal insufficiency is often challenging due to its insidious onset and nonspecific clinical features. Routine laboratory parameters may not indicate any abnormalities until adrenal reserve is critically reduced. However, identification of adrenal insufficiency in a timely manner is crucial in the prevention of adrenal crisis, specifically in high-risk patients undergoing stress (**Figure 4**) [7–9, 12].

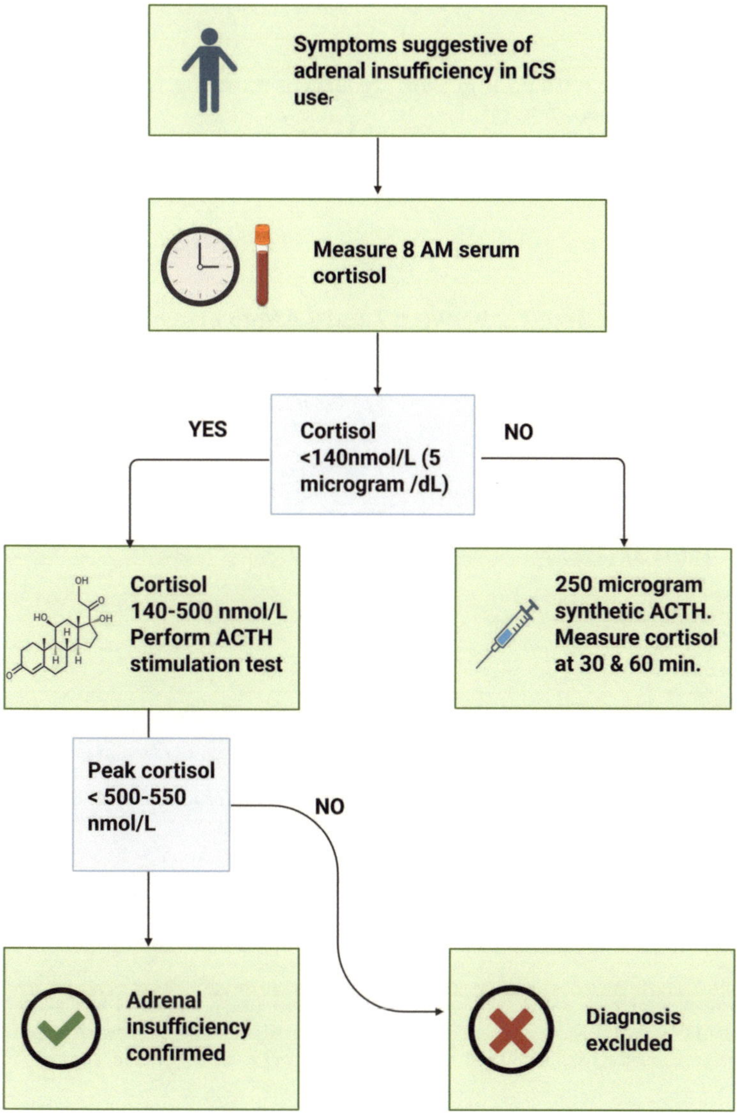

Figure 4.
Diagnosis of ICS induced adrenal insufficiency. Created in BioRender. Cherian [19, 20] https://BioRender.com/rft2wev.

6.1 When should we suspect ICS-induced AI?

1. Use of moderate to high dose ICS for prolonged periods of time

   For example, ≥500mcg/day fluticasone for ≥3 months [10, 16, 17].

2. Simultaneous use of other corticosteroids (topical/ oral)

3. Concurrent administration of CYP3A4 inhibitors (e.g., ketoconazole, ritonavir) [5, 10]

4. Signs of cortisol deficiency: fatigue, nausea, postural hypotension, and hypoglycemia [2, 3]

5. Pediatric patients with poor growth, recurrent morning vomiting, or adrenal crisis during illness [7, 8, 11].

6.2 Baseline morning serum cortisol levels

6.2.1 Timing

Serum cortisol level is tested between **7 and 8 AM** to match the circadian peak (**Table 2**) [2–4].
(Reports can be falsely normal in early stages of HPA axis suppression)

6.3 ACTH stimulation testing

The gold standard test for confirming HPA axis suppression is the short synacthen test (SST) (**Table 3**) [1–3, 7].

Serum Cortisol	Interpretation
>500 nmol/L	Normal HPA function likely
141–500 nmol/L	Indeterminate; further testing needed
<140 nmol/L	Strongly suggestive of adrenal insufficiency

Table 2.
Interpretation of baseline serum cortisol levels.

Protocol	Interpretation
Administer 250 ug synthetic ACTH (cosyntropin) IV or IM. Measure serum cortisol at baseline, 30 and 60 minutes.	Adequate response: peak cortisol >500 nmol/ L Inadequate response: suggests adrenal suppression. In children or partial suppression: 1 ug low-dose test may be more sensitive.

Table 3.
ACTH stimulation testing.

6.4 Additional investigations (optional)

- *ACTH level*: Differentiates between primary and secondary AI
- *DHEA-S*: Decreased in chronic ACTH suppression
- *Electrolytes*: Hyponatremia
- *Glucose*: mild hypoglycemia
- *Bone age X-ray*: in pediatric cases with growth delay [7, 11]
- *Growth velocity and Tanner staging*: in children

7. Pediatric considerations

Due to the body surface area to weight ratio of a child, the evolving HPA axis, and extended potential exposure during critical growth phases, children and adolescents are at a higher risk of experiencing the systemic impacts of inhaled corticosteroids (ICS). Pediatric patients may experience adrenal suppression as a side effect of low to moderate doses of ICS, especially when combined with stronger corticosteroids like fluticasone propionate or budesonide [2, 3, 5–7, 9–12, 16, 17].

7.1 Clinical features in pediatrics

The clinical presentation may be subtle and tends to be nonspecific in nature;

- Increased tiredness, weakness, fatigue, decreased appetite.
- Deceleration in growth or delayed in the onset of puberty [7, 16].
- Head and abdominal pain.
- Low blood sugar, especially during changes in health status.
- Episodes of nonspecific vomiting.

7.2 Screening and monitoring

Screening is indicated for the following patients [7, 11]:

- Children prescribed with high-dose ICS for a duration of three or more months.
- Any child exhibiting suggestive symptoms, regardless of dose.
- Patients transitioning from oral to inhaled corticosteroids [5, 6, 9].

8. Management of ICS-induced adrenal suppression

The management of adrenal insufficiency (AI) due to inhaled corticosteroids depends on the severity of HPA axis suppression, the presence or risk of adrenal crisis, and the necessity of continued corticosteroid therapy for respiratory disease. It requires a balance between minimizing glucocorticoid exposure and preventing life-threatening cortisol deficiency [2, 3, 5–9, 12, 22].

8.1 General principles

1. Identify and discontinue unnecessary corticosteroid exposure (including nasal sprays or topical agents).

2. Taper ICS gradually (if suppression is suspected and the patient is asymptomatic).

3. Educate patients and families on stress dosing and adrenal crisis prevention [7, 8].

4. Initiate hydrocortisone replacement if biochemical or clinical evidence of AI is present [1, 7].

8.2 Glucocorticoid replacement

For patients with confirmed AI:

- Hydrocortisone is favored since it has a short half-life [1, 7].
- The usual dose for adults is 15–25 mg/day in 2–3 doses.
- The usual dose for children is 8–10 mg/m^2/day.
- In places with few resources, prednisolone 3–5 mg/day or cortisone acetate can be used instead.

Mineralocorticoid replacement is unnecessary in ICS-induced (secondary) adrenal insufficiency, as aldosterone secretion remains intact.

8.3 Stress dose education

Patients with adrenal suppression should be educated about stress doses, especially before:

- Surgery
- Severe illness (Example: febrile illnesses or gastroenteritis)
- Trauma or burns.

Protocol for stress dosing:

- Mild illness: double the daily dosage

- Moderate stress (fever >38.5°C): triple dose for 2–3 days
- Surgery or a major illness: 50–100 mg/m^2/day of IV hydrocortisone in divided doses [1, 7].

Children and caregivers must be educated on:

- Emergency administration of hydrocortisone [1, 7]
- Utilization of medical alert bracelets
- Possession of a steroid emergency card.

8.4 Tapering inhaled corticosteroids

ICS should be slowly reduced to allow HPA axis recovery [1–3, 5–7, 9]:

- Taper by 25–50% every 2–4 weeks
- Switch to budesonide or beclomethasone (as they pose lower systemic risk) [9, 12, 16, 17]
- Use spacers and the best technique to keep oropharyngeal deposition to a minimum
- Check clinical state and cortisol levels periodically [2, 3].

In several instances, recuperation transpires within 6–12 months following cessation or dose reduction; however, certain patients may necessitate extended follow-up.

8.5 Monitor recovery

To check the HPA axis's recovery, you should do the following [1, 7]

- Test cortisol levels in the morning every 3–6 months [2, 3].
- Do ACTH stimulation testing again if cortisol levels are higher than 10 µg/dL and the patient is not showing any symptoms [1–3, 7].
- Check children's growth every 3–6 months (height velocity, weight, Tanner staging).

9. Current guidelines and clinical recommendations

There is no universal international consensus guideline specifically addressing inhaled corticosteroid–induced adrenal insufficiency (ICS-AI); however, several expert organizations—including the Endocrine Society, Canadian Pediatric Society (CPS), and European guidelines—offer clinical frameworks that can be modified for risk identification, screening, and management [1, 7, 9, 11, 12].

9.1 Endocrine Society (2016)

The Endocrine Society's guidelines for primary adrenal insufficiency [1, 23] provide recommendations that applies to both iatrogenic and secondary causes, such as ICS-induced suppression [1, 11]:

- Monitor HPA axis functioning in high-risk patients that are on long-term or high-dose steroid exposure, including ICS [2, 3, 9, 12].
- Use the morning serum cortisol test as the first test and the ACTH stimulation test to confirm the results [1–3, 7].
- If suppression is proven, start physiologic hydrocortisone replacement and conduct stress-dose education [1, 7].
- Steadily lower the dose of exogenous corticosteroids (Nasal, oral, or topical) to give the adrenal glands time to recover.

9.2 Canadian pediatric society

The CPS recommends screening and monitoring for adrenal suppression in children taking ICS, especially when [7, 11]:

- The daily dose of ICS is ≥500 mcg of fluticasone (or an equivalent) [10, 16, 17].
- There is more than one type of corticosteroids being utilized (e.g., Nasal, oral, or topical in addition to ICS).
- Children exhibit signs indicative of adrenal insufficiency.
- There is notable growth deceleration.

9.2.1 Important suggestions

- All kids on ICS should have annual growth monitoring.
- Test morning cortisol levels in kids who are at risk for developing AI [2, 3, 9, 12].
- Start hydrocortisone coverage when children are sick or undergoing stress [1, 7].
- Educate families on how to identify clinical features of adrenal crisis and provide them with injectable hydrocortisone if required [1, 7, 8].

9.3 UK medicines and healthcare products regulatory agency (MHRA) alert

The MHRA has issued advisories warning about life-threatening adrenal crises connected to fluticasone, especially in children. They recommend [10, 16, 17]:

- Clinicians should be aware that ICS can have systemic effects, including AI.
- Patients using large doses of fluticasone (more than 500 mcg/day) should be closely monitored for adrenal suppression [10, 16, 17].

- Families should have written information about the indicators of adrenal crisis and when to get immediate help [7, 8].

9.4 Practical clinical recommendations

See **Table 4**.

Domain	Recommendation
Screening	Monitor serum cortisol levels in the morning for patients on >500 mcg/day of ICS for >3 months.
Diagnosis	If cortisol levels are borderline/ low - > confirm with ACTH stimulation test
Management	• Initiate Hydrocortisone administration for confirmed AI. • Educate patients about stress dosing.
Education	Provide patients and families with an adrenal insufficiency action plan
ICS Dosing	Use lowest effective ICS dose to control respiratory symptoms
Technique	Use spacers and proper inhaler technique to reduce systemic absorption
Follow-Up	Reassess HPA axis every 3–6 months during taper or after ICS withdrawal

Table 4.
Practical clinical recommendations.

9.5 Clinical gaps and need for agreement

Even if ICS is widely used, there is:

- No universal standard for evaluating patients that are asymptomatic.
- Not enough information about the threshold doses for testing
- Inconsistent routine monitoring in primary care.

This underscores the necessity for heightened awareness and consistent standards across several specialties—especially in general medicine, pediatrics, pulmonology, and endocrinology (**Table 5**) [7, 11].

Risk category	ICS Dose	Recommendations
Low Risk	< 500 mcg/day fluticasone or equivalent	Use lowest effective dose
Medium Risk	500–1000 mcg/day fluticasone or equivalent	• Monitor for signs of adrenal insufficiency • Annual growth monitoring in children
High Risk	>1000 mcg/day fluticasone or equivalent	• Morning cortisol and/or ACTH stimulation testing • Hydrocortisone for confirmed adrenal insufficiency • Stress dose education

Table 5.
Risk stratification for ICS induced adrenal insufficiency.

10. Prevention strategies

Preventing adrenal suppression with inhaled corticosteroids (ICS) is a very important goal, especially for people who are at risk such as pediatric population, patients on multiple medications, and people who need long-term treatment. To stop this from occurring, you need to limit systemic steroid exposure, make sure you use your inhaler correctly, and raise awareness among both patients and healthcare providers (**Figure 5**) [5–7, 9, 11, 12].

10.1 Use the lowest effective ICS dose

- Adjust the dose until you reach the lowest level that keeps asthma or COPD under control.
- Do not raise the dose too much or use it for too long.
- Every 3 to 6 months, check the ICS dose again, especially in patients who are stable. Research indicates that numerous individuals persist on excessive dosages despite effectively managed respiratory symptoms.

10.2 Improve the way you deliver

- Use spacers with metered-dose inhalers (MDIs) to lower the amount of drug that gets into the oropharynx and the body as a whole.
- Teach patients how to use their inhalers correctly and make sure they remember at every visit.
- After each dose, rinse your mouth and spit to lower the amount of steroid that gets into your mouth and stomach.

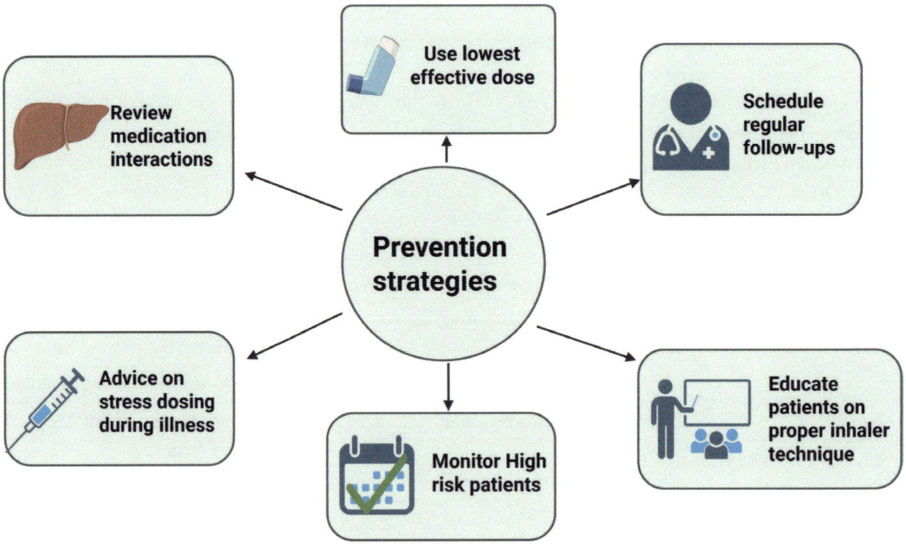

Figure 5.
Methods of prevention of ICS-induced adrenal suppression. Created in BioRender. Cherian [14, 24] https://BioRender.com/qky7xgb.

10.3 Pick ICS formulations

- Choose medicines with lower systemic bioavailability, like budesonide or beclomethasone, especially for children [16, 17].
- Be cautious with fluticasone and ciclesonide as they are powerful and lipophilic ICS, which makes them more likely to cause suppression [25]. The choice of formulation has a big effect on the HPA axis, even when the clinical doses are the same [2, 3, 10, 16, 17].

10.4 Cut down on polypharmacy and interactions

- Do not use more than one type of corticosteroid (for example, ICS + nasal + topical + oral) [7, 11].
- Check for CYP3A4 inhibitors (such ritonavir, itraconazole, and clarithromycin) that slow down ICS metabolism and make the effects on the whole body stronger [5, 10].
- If patients need these drugs, check on them more often or change the ICS choice or dose as needed.

10.5 Proactive monitoring of high-risk patients

Proactive monitoring can help find HPA suppression before it leads to clinical signs or development of a crisis (**Table 6**) [9, 12]:

10.6 Teaching patients and caregivers

- Tell them about the dangers of adrenal suppression, even with inhaled drugs.
- Give a steroid emergency card and detailed instructions for how to dose for stress.
- For children- get school workers and caregivers to help spot indicators of an impending adrenal crisis [7, 8].
- Make sure that emergency hydrocortisone is available if suppression is verified [1, 7].

Risk factors	Monitoring action
ICS dose >500 mcg/day of fluticasone	Morning cortisol every 6 months
Polypharmacy (ICS + other forms of corticosteroids)	• Educate patients • Screen serum cortisol levels every 3–6 months
Pediatric age group (< 12 years)	• Annual growth • Cortisol if symptomatic
CYP3A4 inhibitors	Monitor even at low ICS doses

Table 6.
Guidelines for regular patient monitoring.

10.7 Make prevention a part of everyday care

- Include an ICS risk assessment in the templates for asthma and COPD reviews [9, 12].
- Include growth charts and cortisol tests in visits for kids with asthma [2, 3].
- Use clinical checklists or EMR reminders to keep an eye on high-dose ICS.

11. Conclusion

The use of inhaled corticosteroids is critical for controlling asthma and other chronic respiratory diseases. Nevertheless, there is mounting proof that even these "topical" therapies may disrupt the HPA (Hypothalamic-Pituitary-Adrenal) axis. Adrenal insufficiency (AI) is a condition that is often asymptomatic but poses a significant risk for children, users of high doses of the medication, or those taking it alongside other corticosteroids or enzyme inhibitors [5, 6, 9, 12].

In children, symptoms of tiredness, weight loss, and poor growth make detection difficult. In ICS-induced adrenal insufficiency that is left untreated, there is a risk of progressing toward an adrenal crisis when exposed to physiological stress, which can be life-threatening. Investigation determines diagnosis through morning cortisol levels and ACTH stimulation tests, particularly in defined high-risk populations. Treatment consists of physiologic dose glucocorticoid substitution, education on stress dose teaching, and, where possible, ICS dose reduction [1–3, 7–9, 12].

Most effective is prevention. This includes limiting the ICS to the lowest effective dose, improving inhaler technique, avoiding polypharmacy, and close monitoring of at-risk patients. They particularly aim to lower the dangers while retaining the benefits of ICS therapy [7, 9, 11, 12].

Conflict of interest

The authors declare no conflict of interest..

DOI: http://dx.doi.org/10.5772/intechopen.1012711

Author details

Esha Elizabeth Cherian[1] and Jubbin Jagan Jacob[2*]

1 Dayanand Medical College and Hospital, Ludhiana, Punjab, India

2 Christian Medical College and Hospital, Ludhiana, Punjab, India

*Address all correspondence to: jubbin.jacob@gmail.com

References

[1] Bornstein SR, Allolio B, Arlt W, Barthel A, Don-Wauchope A, Hammer GD, et al. Diagnosis and treatment of primary adrenal insufficiency: An endocrine society clinical practice guideline. The Journal of Clinical Endocrinology and Metabolism. 2016;**101**(2):364-389. DOI: 10.1210/jc.2015-1710

[2] Charmandari E, Nicolaides NC, Chrousos GP. Adrenal insufficiency. Lancet. 2014;**383**(9935):2152-2167. DOI: 10.1016/S0140-6736(13)61684-0. (Open PDF)

[3] Nicolaides NC, Charmandari E, Chrousos GP, Kino T. The hypothalamic–pituitary–adrenal axis and its actions. Annals of the New York Academy of Sciences. 2014;**1318**:1-13

[4] O'Byrne NA, Yuen F, Liu PY. Sleep and circadian regulation of cortisol: A short review. Current Opinion in Endocrine and Metabolic Research. 2021;**16**:100247

[5] Daley-Yates PT. Inhaled corticosteroids: Potency, dose equivalence and therapeutic index. British Journal of Clinical Pharmacology. 2015;**80**(3):372-380

[6] Pandya D, Puttanna A, Balagopal V. Systemic effects of inhaled corticosteroids: An overview. Open Respiratory Medicine Journal. 2014;**8**:59-65. Open access

[7] Ahmet A, Kim H, Spier S. Adrenal suppression: A practical guide to the screening and management of this under-recognized complication of inhaled corticosteroid therapy. Allergy, Asthma and Clinical Immunology. 2011;7(1):13

[8] Hay CM, Henley DE, Talbot DC, et al. Adrenal insufficiency in a woman secondary to standard-dose inhaled fluticasone propionate therapy. Journal of Medical Case Reports. 2014;**8**:93

[9] Patel R, Hurst JR, Van Staa T, et al. Systemic adverse effects from inhaled corticosteroid use in asthma: A systematic review and meta-analysis. BMJ Open Respiratory Research. 2020;7(1):e000756. Open access

[10] UK MHRA. Drug Safety Update: Interactions between CYP3A-metabolised corticosteroids and HIV pharmacokinetic boosters—risk of adrenal suppression. December 2016. (Regulatory safety advisory; open PDF)

[11] Hossny E, Caraballo L, Casale T, et al. The use of inhaled corticosteroids in pediatric asthma: Update. World Allergy Organization Journal. 2016;**9**:26

[12] Lee H, Jang S, Kim SR, et al. Inhaled corticosteroid increased the risk of adrenal insufficiency in patients with chronic airway diseases: A nationwide cohort study. Scientific Reports. 2024;**14**:15264. Open access

[13] Herman JP, McKlveen JM, Ghosal S, Kopp B, Wulsin A, Makinson R, et al. Regulation of the hypothalamic-pituitary-adrenocortical stress response. Comprehensive Physiology. 2016;**6**(2):603-621

[14] Cherian E. Physiology of the Hypothalamic–Pituitary–Adrenal Axis. Toronto (ON): BioRender; 2025. Available from: https://BioRender.com/qky7xgb

[15] Cherian E. Pharmacokinetics and Pharmacodynamics of Inhaled

Corticosteroids. Toronto (ON): BioRender; 2025. Available from: https://BioRender.com/o0wov2g

[16] Ahmet A, Benchimol EI, Goldbloom EB, et al. Adrenal suppression in children treated with swallowed fluticasone and oral viscous budesonide for eosinophilic esophagitis. Allergy, Asthma and Clinical Immunology. 2016;**12**:49. Open access

[17] Sannarangappa V, Jalleh R. Inhaled corticosteroids and secondary adrenal insufficiency. Open Respiratory Medicine Journal. 2014;**8**:93-100. Open access

[18] Gutiérrez LS, Zorrilla AM, Quiroga MV, et al. Iatrogenic Cushing syndrome and secondary adrenal insufficiency due to inhaled fluticasone. Cureus. 2021;**13**(4):e14405

[19] Cherian E. Pathophysiology of ICS-Induced Adrenal Insufficiency. Toronto (ON): BioRender; 2025. Available from: https://BioRender.com/rft2wev

[20] Cherian E. Diagnosis of ICS-Induced Adrenal Insufficiency—Algorithm. Toronto (ON): BioRender; 2025. Available from: https://BioRender.com/rft2wev

[21] NIDDK. Secondary adrenal insufficiency—definition & facts. (Patient-facing physiology explainer; useful for plain-language boxes)

[22] Heffler E, Madeira LNG, Ferrando M, et al. Inhaled corticosteroids safety and adverse effects in patients with asthma. The Journal of Allergy and Clinical Immunology. In Practice. 2018;**6**(3):776-781. (Good overview; abstract public)

[23] Endocrine Society. Primary adrenal insufficiency guideline resources (practice points & patient safety); 2016

[24] Cherian E. Prevention of ICS-Induced Adrenal Suppression. Toronto (ON): BioRender; 2025. Available from: https://BioRender.com/qky7xgb

[25] GSK (Fluticasone propionate inhalation aerosol, FLOBENT/Flovent) Product Monograph. 2021. (Label statements on HPA suppression and crisis risk; open PDF)

Chapter 6

Corticosteroid Therapy in Rheumatology: Essential Treatment, Challenges and Solutions

Cristina Criveanu

Abstract

This chapter emphasizes the therapeutic role of corticosteroids in rheumatic diseases, underlining their importance in suppressing inflammation and alleviating symptoms. Corticosteroids serve as key agents in the control of rheumatic diseases, with their anti-inflammatory action proving valuable in conditions such as rheumatoid arthritis, systemic lupus erythematosus, and polymyalgia rheumatica. Although they have significant therapeutic effects, long-term use of corticosteroids involves significant risks, such as osteoporosis, hypertension, and diabetes, which generate challenges in patient management. This chapter analyzes strategies for optimizing corticosteroid treatment, including dose adjustment, the use of rescue therapy, and association with other drugs to minimize side effects. The chapter also discusses strategies aimed at enhancing patients' quality of life and reducing long-term complications, including continuous monitoring and multidisciplinary care. Its objective is to provide deeper insight into the role of corticosteroids in rheumatology, emphasizing the balance between therapeutic benefits and potential risks.

Keywords: rheumatology, corticotherapy, adverse effects, rheumatic diseases, inflammation

1. Introduction

1.1 Historical perspective of corticosteroid use in rheumatology

Glucocorticoid therapy remains a most often life-saving therapy in patients with inflammatory rheumatic diseases, despite all major developments in rheumatic disease therapies.

Until the first half of the twentieth century, conditions associated with adrenal insufficiency, such as Addison's disease, did not benefit from effective treatments, unlike hypothyroidism, where the administration of thyroid extracts quickly proved beneficial [1].

In 1930, biochemists Wilbur W. Swingle and Joseph J. Pfiffner of Princeton University succeeded in extracting a limited amount of the active substance from the adrenal cortex, sufficient for the first clinical trials. The process was extremely laborious: it was necessary to process the adrenal glands of two bulls to obtain a single milliliter of injectable product [2].

At the Mayo Clinic, under the direction of Leonard G. Rowntree, clinical trials were conducted on patients with Addison's disease and other patients, using doses of 40–60 ml administered intravenously over 4–10 days. The effects were only transient. The impact was only temporary. Swingle and Pfiffner's technique was subsequently taken up and refined by additional teams of investigators. The starting material consisted of 3–4 kg of bovine adrenal glands, frozen immediately after slaughter. The extraction process involved finely chopping the tissue and using successive solvents (ethanol and acetone), with an essential step of removing epinephrine. The final product was an extract generically called "cortin", a term first used by F.A. Hartman in 1928, suggesting the existence of an active cortical hormone [3].

Beginning in the 1930s, Edward C. Kendall at the Mayo Clinic and Tadeus Reichstein in Zurich [4] led crucial efforts to purify and characterize adrenocortical compounds. In December 1933, a compound – initially named *compound E*, which was later named *cortisone* was obtained in crystalline form, paving the way for its synthesis and widespread therapeutic use [4].

1.2 Rationale and scope of corticosteroid therapy

The history of rheumatology reached a pivotal moment on April 13, 1949, when the *Proceedings of the Staff Meetings* of the Mayo Clinic published the first account of cortisone therapy in a patient with rheumatoid arthritis [5]. This pioneering work was directed by Philip S. Hench, who served as Chief of the Division of Rheumatology at the Mayo Clinic. The initial case involved a 29-year-old woman with a four-year history of severe rheumatoid arthritis (RA) that had not responded to the conventional therapies available at that time. Before the administration of cortisone, she had been treated at the Mayo Clinic since February 1948, without achieving significant disease control.

The protocol followed the dosing regimen previously used in experimental tests with "Compound A". Starting on September 21, 1948, the patient received intramuscular injections of 50 mg of cortisone twice a day. After the second injection, a significant subjective improvement was reported. After 9 days, the dosage was lowered to 50 mg per day and subsequently to 25 mg; however, by day 17, the musculoskeletal symptoms had worsened. Resumption of the initial regimen (50 mg twice a day) improved the symptoms again. After 23 days of treatment, visible side effects appeared – facial edema (puffy face). At 60 days of treatment, the patient developed facial hirsutism, acne, psychiatric disorders, depressive thinking, hostility, and emotional instability. However, rheumatic symptoms were reported to be improved by approximately 50%. No withdrawal symptoms or discontinuation syndrome were noted at the time of discharge in May 1949 [6]. This case marked the beginning of the clinical use of cortisone in rheumatology, highlighting both its remarkable therapeutic potential and its significant adverse reaction profile, especially with prolonged administration or at high doses. The event spurred continued research, which rapidly facilitated the extensive application of synthetic glucocorticoids in managing autoimmune and inflammatory diseases.

The outstanding therapeutic impact of cortisone in rheumatoid arthritis and other inflammatory conditions quickly drew worldwide scientific recognition. The Nobel Prize in Physiology or Medicine for 1950 was presented collectively to three distinguished figures:

- Philip S. Hench, for demonstrating the clinical benefits of cortisone in rheumatology, particularly in rheumatoid arthritis.
- Edward C. Kendall, for isolating and chemically characterizing the adrenal cortex compound initially termed Compound E, later identified as cortisone.
- Tadeus Reichstein – for his contributions to the elucidation of the structure and partial synthesis of the adrenocortical hormones.

This recognition marked the beginning of the era of modern hormonal therapies in systemic inflammatory diseases. The award highlighted the value of collaboration between basic research (chemistry and biochemistry) and clinical practice, demonstrating how laboratory discoveries can transform the treatment of diseases previously considered disabling or progressive. It further opened the path to the creation of cortisone derivatives, designed with enhanced pharmacological activity and improved safety characteristics.

2. Mechanism of action and pharmacological properties

2.1 Glucocorticoid receptors and molecular pathways

Glucocorticoids (GCs) exert their complex biological effects by binding to specific intracellular receptors, followed by the activation of molecular cascades with an essential role in the regulation of inflammation, metabolism, and immunological homeostasis.

At the cellular level, the actions of glucocorticoids are primarily mediated by an intracellular receptor protein known as the glucocorticoid receptor (GR). The gene encoding this receptor is designated NR3C1 (nuclear receptor subfamily 3, group C, member 1), and it belongs to the extensive nuclear receptor superfamily, which includes over 200 members across species and more than 40 cloned and characterized members in mammals [7]. As a ligand-activated transcription factor, the glucocorticoid receptor (GR) is organized in a modular fashion, including

- N-terminal transactivation domain (NTD): plays a role in regulating transcriptional activity.
- DNA-binding domain (DBD): enables the receptor to attach to specific DNA sequences known as glucocorticoid response elements (GREs). N-terminal transactivation domain (NTD) – involved in modulating transcriptional activity.
- Hinge region – provides flexibility to the receptor.
- Ligand-binding domain (LBD) – where glucocorticoids interact with the receptor.

Two major isoforms of GR are recognized:

- GRα is the classical 777-amino acid isoform that mediates the canonical anti-inflammatory and immunomodulatory effects of glucocorticoids. It achieves this through ligand binding, nuclear translocation, and regulation of gene transcription, serving as the active form that transduces the biological actions of glucocorticoids.

- GRβ is a shorter, 742-amino acid isoform produced through alternative splicing at exon 9. Acting as a dominant-negative variant, it may contribute to reduced glucocorticoid responsiveness, especially in the setting of autoimmune and inflammatory diseases.

The sequences of GRα and GRβ are identical through amino acid 727; however, GRβ contains a unique C-terminal segment, resulting in a shortened ligand-binding domain (LBD) that lacks helix 12 [8].

Due to this structural alteration, GRβ cannot bind endogenous glucocorticoids, yet it is constitutively localized in the nucleus where it exerts distinct biological functions. GRβ has been reported to compete with GRα for binding to glucocorticoid response elements (GREs) as well as for common co-regulatory proteins [9]. Additionally, form inactive GRα/GRβ heterodimers, attenuating the overall glucocorticoid response. It regulates a unique set of genes independent of both GRα and glucocorticoid ligands, expanding its functional repertoire beyond antagonism [9–11]. Interestingly, GRβ, although unresponsive to endogenous glucocorticoids, demonstrates binding affinity for certain synthetic antagonists, such as RU-486 (mifepristone), suggesting that selective synthetic ligands could modulate GRβ activity in the future.

Glucocorticoid production is tightly regulated by the hypothalamic-pituitary-adrenal (HPA) axis, essential for physiological homeostasis. In a normal state, GCs enter the bloodstream following circadian and ultradian rhythms, peaking in humans in the morning and in nocturnal species during early night. In response to physiological or emotional stress, the hypothalamus releases corticotropin-releasing hormone (CRH) and arginine vasopressin (AVP). These molecules activate CRH-R1 and V1B receptors in the anterior pituitary, resulting in the secretion of adrenocorticotropic hormone (ACTH), which stimulates the adrenal glands to produce cortisol, the primary glucocorticoid in humans [12].

Through negative feedback, cortisol suppresses gene transcription in both the hypothalamus and pituitary, targeting CRH, CRH-R1, and POMC (the ACTH precursor) [13–15]. This occurs *via* binding of glucocorticoid receptors (GRs) to negative glucocorticoid response elements (nGREs) and through direct modulation of the transcription factor Nur77, which governs POMC expression [16, 17]. Glucocorticoids passively diffuse into the cell, bind cytoplasmic GRs, and form a complex that migrates to the nucleus to influence transcription [18, 19].

There are two major pathways by which this complex modulates gene expression:

Transactivation: The glucocorticoid-GR complex binds to specific DNA sequences called glucocorticoid response elements (GREs), stimulating the transcription of anti-inflammatory genes such as lipocortin-1, IL-10, and decoy receptors [20]. It also mediates *transrepression* by interfering with proinflammatory transcription factors like NFκB and AP-1, thereby inhibiting the production of cytokines, chemokines, adhesion molecules, and enzymes involved in inflammatory responses [21]. Genomic effects typically occur 30–60 minutes after administration, requiring time for transcription and protein translation.

There are also non-genomic mechanisms of regulation of the HPA axis: release of endocannabinoids by CRH neurons, reducing excitatory glutamatergic transmission [22], stimulation of GABA release, enhancing synaptic inhibition of CRH neurons [23], modification of membrane fluidity and direct interaction with membrane proteins, activation or inhibition of cytoplasmatic signaling cascades such as MAPK, PI3K or ion channels [24]. The non-genomic actions of glucocorticoids occur within seconds to minutes and function independently of GR movement into the nucleus and transcriptional regulation. These effects are particularly relevant in emergency situations, such as septic shock or acute exacerbations of autoimmune diseases, where rapid improvements are observed following glucocorticoid therapy.

2.2 Pharmacokinetics and pharmacodynamics

The pharmacokinetic profile of glucocorticoids depends on their physicochemical properties. After oral intake, glucocorticoids demonstrate good absorption and a bioavailability of around 60–100%. Intravenous administration is also common, especially in acute settings. The agents show a moderate degree of plasma protein binding and a correspondingly moderate apparent volume of distribution.

The pharmacokinetics of hydrocortisone (cortisol) and prednisolone are nonlinear, mainly as a result of their binding interactions with plasma proteins. Both drugs bind to transcortin (also known as corticosteroid-binding globulin, CBG) and albumin. While transcortin demonstrates high-affinity, limited-capacity binding, albumin binds with low affinity but high capacity. At lower plasma concentrations, most of the glucocorticoid is bound to transcortin. Once transcortin becomes saturated, usually at plasma concentrations around 400 μg/L-further increases in glucocorticoid levels lead to a greater fraction of the hormone remaining unbound (free). This saturation effect is commonly observed after administration of hydrocortisone or prednisolone doses exceeding 20 mg, leading to a nonlinear increase in the free, active fraction of the drug [25]. Although these lipophilic agents are efficiently absorbed, significant first-pass metabolism may limit their oral bioavailability, rendering them suboptimal for systemic oral use while favoring topical and inhaled routes.

The pharmacokinetic profile of different types of glucocorticoids differs significantly depending on their potency, duration of action, and biochemical properties.

Prednisone is a potent synthetic glucocorticoid, commonly used in medical practice for its anti-inflammatory and immunosuppressive effects. From a pharmacokinetic point of view, prednisone is a prodrug, meaning that it is not biologically active immediately after administration. After oral administration, prednisone is absorbed from the gastrointestinal tract, with a bioavailability of approximately 70–90% [26, 27]. Once absorbed, it undergoes enzymatic reduction in the liver to form its active metabolite, prednisolone. Prednisone itself has a relatively short plasma half-life of about 1 hour, whereas prednisolone exhibits a half-life of 2–4 hours [25, 26]. However, the biological effect of prednisolone lasts longer than its plasma half-life, extending over a period of about 12–36 hours. The liver is the main site of prednisone metabolism, and its metabolites are primarily eliminated through renal excretion in an inactive state. Prednisone has mild mineralocorticoid activity and is frequently used in inflammatory and autoimmune diseases or in replacement therapy.

Methylprednisolone is a synthetic glucocorticoid with a potency similar to prednisolone, but with significantly reduced mineralocorticoid activity, making it preferred in certain pathologies where sodium and water retention must be avoided [28]. Administered orally or intravenously, methylprednisolone has very good absorption, with a bioavailability of over 80–90% [29]. Unlike prednisone, methylprednisolone does not require hepatic activation, being biologically active immediately after absorption. While the plasma half-life is around 2–3 hours, the drug's therapeutic effects can last between 12 and 36 hours. It is 70–80% bound to plasma proteins, mainly to transcortin and albumin [30]. Methylprednisolone is metabolized in the liver and predominantly eliminated *via* the kidneys as inactive metabolites. There are also injectable preparations of methylprednisolone, such as methylprednisolone succinate, which is frequently used in medical emergencies, such as severe allergic reactions or exacerbations of autoimmune diseases [31].

Dexamethasone is a synthetic glucocorticoid characterized by high potency and a markedly longer duration of action than prednisone or methylprednisolone. After oral administration, dexamethasone is well absorbed, with a bioavailability of approximately 70–78% [32]. Being biologically active in the administered form, it does not require prior hepatic conversion. Dexamethasone exhibits a plasma half-life of about 3–5 hours, yet its pharmacological effects may last 36–72 hours, classifying it as a long-acting glucocorticoid [33]. It is less bound to plasma proteins than the other glucocorticoids, approximately 65%, which means that a significant fraction remains free and active in the circulation. An important aspect is that dexamethasone has negligible mineralocorticoid activity, which makes it useful in treatments where sodium and water retention must be avoided, such as in cerebral edema or various severe inflammatory conditions. Similar to other glucocorticoids, dexamethasone undergoes hepatic metabolism and is primarily excreted by the kidneys as inactive metabolites.

3. Clinical applications in rheumatologic disorders

3.1 Glucocorticoids in rheumatoid arthritis

Shortly after the introduction of cortisone and hydrocortisone in the treatment of rheumatoid arthritis (RA), it was observed that these corticosteroids undergo interconversion processes *in vivo*, and the activity of the enzyme 11β-hydroxysteroid dehydrogenase (11β-HSD) is essential for the conversion of cortisone to cortisol [34]. This finding led to the hypothesis that synovial tissue might have the capacity to metabolize corticosteroids locally. Initially, it was assumed that patients with RA would have an increased capacity to inactivate hydrocortisone [35].

Although, at that time, the understanding of the processes of corticosteroid metabolism at the tissue level was limited, the existence of a bidirectional activity of the enzyme 11β-HSD in the synovial tissue affected by RA was demonstrated [36], and subsequent studies showed that the injection of cortisone directly into the inflamed joints leads to the generation of significant amounts of cortisol locally [37].

Recent research has renewed interest in this area, particularly because 11β-HSD2 isoenzyme expression appears to contribute to RA development. In peripheral blood mononuclear cells (PBMCs) from patients with newly diagnosed rheumatoid arthritis, 11β-HSD2 emerged as the most abundantly expressed gene among over 4300 genes analyzed, relative to patients with long-standing disease [38]. Histological analyses of synovial tissue have shown that 11β-HSD2 expression is predominantly localized to synovial macrophages. Another study evaluating the ability of synovial explants to inactivate corticosteroids indicated significantly increased metabolic activity in RA patients [39]. That investigation did not directly measure glucocorticoid activation but rather used 11β-HSD inhibitors, which lack full specificity. In addition, the connection between tissue-specific and systemic glucocorticoid metabolism has yet to be adequately clarified. In order to clarify these aspects, studies using specific enzyme activity assays and selective inhibitors of the enzymes involved have been performed to accurately define the nature of corticosteroid metabolic pathways. The potential impact of local corticosteroid metabolism on local and systemic glucocorticoid concentrations has also been examined [40].

One of the most appreciated effects of glucocorticoids is that of "bridge therapy", which represents a bridge until disease-modifying drugs take effect in patients with RA. This effect was confirmed by a meta-analysis based on individual patient data, which evaluated extended glucocorticoid therapy after bridging treatment in RA [41]. The study included 1653 patients from seven randomized clinical trials. The results showed that although most patients were able to discontinue glucocorticoids after the bridging period, a significant proportion continued treatment long-term (approximately 30% at 2 years). Factors associated with prolonged use were higher initial doses and extended duration regimens. In conclusion, glucocorticoids should be used as bridging therapy only for a limited duration and at the lowest effective dose, in order to minimize the risks associated with long-term exposure and adverse effects [41].

3.2 Glucocorticoids in systemic lupus erythematosus

Due to their rapid anti-inflammatory and immunosuppressive effects, glucocorticoids are essential for managing acute flares of systemic lupus erythematosus (SLE) and other connective tissue diseases (CTDs). In SLE, they still remain the first-line treatment in organ-threatening manifestations such as neuropsychiatric lupus, lupus nephritis, or severe hematological involvement [42]. Their use allows rapid control of systemic inflammation and prevents the progression of irreversible lesions. Therefore, current therapeutic strategies aim to use the lowest effective dose, in combination with immunomodulatory agents or biological therapies, to minimize chronic exposure [43, 44].

In other BCTs, such as dermatomyositis, scleroderma, or Sjögren's syndrome with systemic involvement, glucocorticoids remain a therapeutic mainstay in acute phases or severe forms, especially when there is significant pulmonary, renal, or muscle involvement [45].

3.3 Vasculitis and inflammatory myopathies

Vasculitis represent a diverse spectrum of diseases in which inflammation of the blood vessel walls can cause impaired perfusion, tissue ischemia, and subsequent organ injury. Glucocorticoids are the mainstay of treatment in most forms of vasculitis, playing an essential role in controlling acute inflammation and preventing tissue destruction [46]. In severe forms, such as microscopic polyangiitis, granulomatosis with polyangiitis (Wegener), treatment usually begins with intravenous methylprednisolone at 500–1000 mg/day for 3 days, after which oral prednisone is administered at 1 mg/kg/day, with doses progressively reduced according to clinical improvement [47].

For conditions like giant cell arteritis, a form of large-vessel vasculitis, glucocorticoids remain the primary treatment, crucial for avoiding severe outcomes, including blindness. Early administration of prednisone (40–60 mg/day) may prevent ocular ischemia and other ischemic complications [48].

In all forms of vasculitis, glucocorticoids are recommended in combination with immunosuppressive agents-such as cyclophosphamide, azathioprine, or methotrexate-or biologic therapies like rituximab, with the goal of limiting long-term corticosteroid exposure and reducing associated risks.

Glucocorticoids are the primary treatment for *inflammatory myopathies*, typically starting with prednisone at 0.5–1 mg/kg/day, adjusted according to the severity of the condition. In severe forms, with respiratory impairment, swallowing dysfunction or myocardial impairment, intravenous pulses of methylprednisolone can be used. The response to therapy is assessed by improving muscle strength and decreasing muscle enzyme levels (CK, LDH, and aldolase). To achieve sustained disease control and reduce the adverse effects of glucocorticoids, immunosuppressive agents (methotrexate, azathioprine) or intravenous immunoglobulins are frequently associated, especially in refractory dermatomyositis or cancer-associated myopathies [49, 50].

3.4 Gout and crystal-induced arthropathies

Glucocorticoids are a key treatment option during acute episodes of gout or exacerbations of crystal-induced arthropathies, especially for patients who cannot tolerate NSAIDs or colchicine, or who have marked renal dysfunction [51].

Glucocorticoid therapy may be adjusted according to both the intensity and the distribution of the joint involvement. Thus, in monoarticular or oligoarticular attacks, intra-articular infiltrations with methylprednisolone or triamcinolone have proven particularly effective, rapidly reducing local inflammation and relieving pain, with a minimal risk of systemic reactions [52]. In contrast, for severe or polyarticular attacks, systemic glucocorticoid therapy is indicated, either orally, with prednisone initiated at 30–40 mg/day and gradually tapered over 7–10 days, or intravenously, using methylprednisolone pulses, particularly in refractory cases or when complex comorbidities are present [53].

Pseudogout, although clinically it can mimic gout attacks, has a distinct pathophysiology, involving calcium pyrophosphate crystal deposition. In this situation, too, glucocorticoids are used successfully, especially in cases with polyarticular manifestations or in elderly patients, where other therapies may present increased risks [54].

From a therapeutic perspective, the three principal drug classes used in gout and crystal-induced arthropathies are glucocorticoids, NSAIDs, and colchicine. Treatment selection is guided by the severity of the attack, the number of joints involved, the patient's safety profile, and coexisting comorbidities [55]. Numerous studies have demonstrated that glucocorticoids have comparable efficacy to NSAIDs in controlling acute gout attacks. For instance, a study conducted by Man et al. found that a five-day course of oral prednisolone (35 mg/day) provided comparable relief from joint pain and inflammation as naproxen 500 mg twice daily, while offering a safer profile, particularly in older adults or individuals with cardiovascular risk factors [56].

3.5 Intra-articular and local glucocorticoid injections

Local and intra-articular corticosteroid administration is a widely used therapeutic approach in rheumatology, aimed at reducing joint inflammation and alleviating pain, especially in inflammatory and degenerative conditions. Local administration achieves a swift anti-inflammatory response concentrated on the targeted structure, minimizing systemic absorption and the potential adverse effects of generalized glucocorticoid therapy [57].

The effectiveness of corticosteroid injections has been well-established in managing synovitis associated with rheumatoid arthritis, crystal-induced arthropathies, osteoarthritis, tenosynovitis, and bursitis. For instance, intra-articular administration of triamcinolone hexacetonide or methylprednisolone acetate often results in substantial pain relief and decreased joint swelling, with therapeutic effects lasting from several weeks to months, depending on disease severity and individual patient response [58, 59].

A major advantage of local injections is the avoidance of undesirable systemic effects, such as hyperglycemia, hypertension, or osteoporosis, especially when repeated doses or prolonged systemic therapy are administered. In addition, infiltration of corticosteroids allows for targeted treatment of joints or periarticular structures that are difficult to approach by other methods, such as inflamed bursae or tendon sheaths [60].

Randomized trials have confirmed the advantages of intra-articular corticosteroid injections, particularly for symptom management in knee osteoarthritis. A meta-analysis by McAlindon et al. showed that such injections provide significant pain relief and functional improvement, although the effects are generally transient, underscoring the need for selective use and careful monitoring [61].

However, frequent and repetitive use of intra-articular injections is not without risks. Reported complications include joint infections (rare but severe), structural joint damage, skin atrophy or skin discoloration at the injection site [62].

4. Adverse effects and risk management

4.1 Metabolic and endocrine complications

The use of glucocorticoids, either systemically or by repeated local administration, is associated with a wide range of metabolic and endocrine complications, which can significantly affect the quality of life of patients and may limit the long-term use of these potent anti-inflammatory agents.

One of the most common and well-documented complications is the induction of hyperglycemia and the aggravation of diabetes mellitus. Glucocorticoids may promote the development of steroid-induced diabetes over time by enhancing gluconeogenesis in the liver, impairing glucose uptake in peripheral tissues, and inducing insulin resistance, especially in patients with existing risk factors [63, 64]. In addition, episodes of hyperglycemia can occur even after intra-articular or inhaled glucocorticoids, especially in elderly patients or patients with pre-existing diabetes [58].

In terms of lipids, glucocorticoids induce dyslipidemia, characterized by increased triglycerides and LDL cholesterol, along with a possible decrease in HDL cholesterol. These changes contribute to increased long-term cardiovascular risk, along with the hypertension frequently associated with glucocorticoid therapy [65].

Another major metabolic effect is the redistribution of body fat, a phenomenon known as "Cushingoid obesity". This is manifested by the accumulation of adipose tissue in the face (round, "moon-shaped" facies), the posterior cervical region ("buffalo neck") and the trunk, with muscle atrophy in the limbs, classic aspects of iatrogenically induced Cushing's syndrome [66].

Glucocorticoids negatively impact bone by altering phospho-calcium homeostasis, inhibiting osteogenesis, promoting bone resorption, and decreasing calcium absorption in the gut. These mechanisms contribute to osteoporosis in chronically treated patients, significantly elevating the risk of vertebral and hip fractures [67, 68].

From an endocrine standpoint, one of the most serious complications of glucocorticoid therapy is suppression of the hypothalamic-pituitary-adrenal (HPA) axis, which can be potentially fatal if high-dose or long-term treatment is abruptly stopped. This suppression leads to secondary adrenal insufficiency, manifested by fatigue, hypotension, hyponatremia or even adrenal crises in acute stress situations [69].

4.2 Osteoporosis and musculoskeletal effects

Glucocorticoid-induced osteoporosis (GIOP) can develop soon after treatment initiation, with bone loss being most pronounced during the first 6–12 months. The risk of vertebral and hip fractures rises even with moderate long-term doses, equivalent to ≥5 mg of prednisone per day [70, 71].

The pathogenic mechanisms are complex and multifactorial, including direct suppression of osteoblast activity and the induction of apoptosis in both osteoblasts and osteocytes, ultimately leading to decreased bone formation. In parallel, glucocorticoids prolong the lifespan of osteoclasts, favoring bone resorption [72]. Glucocorticoid therapy also impairs calcium homeostasis by decreasing intestinal absorption and enhancing renal excretion, resulting in functional hypocalcemia and secondary hyperparathyroidism that accelerate bone loss [73].

Glucocorticoid therapy may also lead to muscle wasting, predominantly in the proximal lower-limb muscles, a phenomenon known as *glucocorticoid-induced myopathy*. This condition is clinically manifested by muscle weakness, fatigue, and reduced mobility, with a negative impact on the patient's functional independence [74].

Up to half of patients on chronic glucocorticoid therapy may develop osteoporosis, and the incidence of asymptomatic vertebral fractures can approach 50% in some groups, influenced by both dose and duration of treatment [75, 76].

International guidelines, including those from the American College of Rheumatology, underscore the importance of fracture risk assessment using tools such as FRAX, performing bone densitometry (DXA), and initiating early preventive measures. These measures encompass calcium and vitamin D supplementation, lifestyle modifications, and, in high-risk patients, the use of antiresorptive therapies such as bisphosphonates [77, 78].

4.3 Cardiovascular and neuropsychiatric effects

Glucocorticoid therapy contributes to cardiovascular risk by promoting hypertension, dyslipidemia, insulin resistance, and atherosclerotic progression, potentially culminating in myocardial infarction or stroke [79, 80]. The mechanisms involved include sodium and water retention through stimulation of mineralocorticoid receptors, increased vascular tone, and impaired lipid and carbohydrate metabolism [81].

Chronic administration of glucocorticoids, especially at medium and high doses, has been linked in observational studies to heightened cardiovascular risk, regardless of traditional risk factors [82]. Furthermore, doses below 10 mg prednisone/day may still promote hypertension or worsen pre-existing hypertension in predisposed patients [83].

Glucocorticoid therapy is also associated with neuropsychiatric effects, which can range widely in severity and presentation and may include mood changes, insomnia, irritability, anxiety, and, in severe cases, psychosis or major depression [84]. These manifestations are generically referred to as "steroid psychosis" and occur more frequently at high doses, but can also occur with long-term administration at moderate doses [85].

Of interest is the association between glucocorticoids and impaired cognitive function, particularly in the elderly, where chronic treatment may contribute to memory impairment or subtle cognitive decline by affecting the hippocampus and other cortisol-sensitive brain structures [86, 87].

The risk of neuropsychiatric adverse effects is influenced by individual factors, including pre-existing vulnerabilities, history of psychiatric disorders, and dosage administered. Symptoms usually resolve with dose reduction or discontinuation, but severe cases require specific psychiatric and/or pharmacological interventions [88].

4.4 Infection risk and immunosuppression

Glucocorticoids increase susceptibility to infections through multiple mechanisms, including inhibition of T and B lymphocyte function, reduced production of proinflammatory cytokines, impaired phagocyte migration and activity, and compromised antiviral responses [89]. In addition, by reducing inflammation and masking classic signs of infection, glucocorticoids may delay the diagnosis and appropriate treatment of already present infections [90].

The risk of infections is influenced by glucocorticoid dose, duration, and route of administration. Observational studies indicate that chronic use of prednisone equivalents exceeding 7.5 mg/day markedly increases the incidence of bacterial, viral, and fungal infections, including pneumonia, opportunistic infections, and viral reactivations such as herpes zoster [91, 92]. Furthermore, the combined use of glucocorticoids with other immunosuppressive agents—such as methotrexate, cyclophosphamide, or tumor necrosis factor (TNF) inhibitors—significantly elevates the cumulative risk of serious infections [93].

Glucocorticoids also increase the risk of reactivated latent tuberculosis, requiring screening and prophylaxis in endemic regions or in patients with personal risk factors [94]. Beyond bacterial and fungal infections, high-dose glucocorticoid therapy has been linked to a higher incidence of severe viral infections, including cytomegalovirus, herpes simplex virus, and serious respiratory infections such as COVID-19 [95].

Considering the well-established risk of infections linked to glucocorticoid therapy, it is essential that the management of these patients includes proactive monitoring and prevention measures. Prevention of infectious complications involves both rigorous evaluation of patients before initiating treatment and ongoing monitoring during therapy [96, 97].

Before starting glucocorticoids, patients-particularly those with previous TB exposure, contact with infected persons, or from endemic areas-should be screened for latent infections, especially tuberculosis.

Assessment of the patient's vaccination status is also recommended. Vaccinations for influenza, pneumococcus, hepatitis B, and varicella-zoster virus should ideally be completed before starting immunosuppressive therapy, since live vaccines cannot be safely given during high-dose glucocorticoid treatment [98, 99].

Careful monitoring of patients receiving glucocorticoids is essential for the timely identification of infections, as these medications may mask typical symptoms like fever and local inflammatory responses [91]. In addition, biological parameters, including the complete blood count and inflammatory markers, should be monitored to detect possible subclinical infections [90].

In the case of prolonged administration or doses equivalent to prednisone >7.5 mg/day, specific prophylaxis against opportunistic infections should be considered. For instance, to mitigate the risk of Pneumocystis jirovecii pneumonia, particularly in patients with severe autoimmune diseases or those receiving concomitant immunosuppressive therapy, prophylaxis with trimethoprim-sulfamethoxazole is recommended [100].

In addition, reducing the risk of infection can be achieved by using the lowest effective dose of glucocorticoids, rapid dose titration, and exploring steroid-sparing treatment options, such as the use of biologic agents or antimetabolites, depending on the underlying pathology [89].

In pandemics or in special epidemiological situations, such as SARS-CoV-2 infection, patients on corticosteroid treatment require additional monitoring, adjustment of immunosuppressive therapy, and, if necessary, full vaccination, taking into account specific indications for immunocompromised patients [95].

5. Alternative and adjunctive therapies

In the management of chronic inflammatory and autoimmune diseases, reducing glucocorticoid dependence is an essential goal, given their extensive adverse effect profile. Alternative or adjunctive strategies include the use of corticosteroid-sparing agents, biologic therapies, small molecules, and nonpharmacological interventions, which contribute to disease control and minimize corticosteroid exposure.

5.1 Corticosteroid-sparing agents

Classical immunosuppressive drugs such as methotrexate, azathioprine, mycophenolate mofetil, and cyclophosphamide are used as corticosteroid-sparing therapies in conditions like systemic lupus erythematosus, vasculitis, and rheumatoid arthritis, allowing glucocorticoid doses to be lowered or stopped while maintaining disease management [101, 102].

Methotrexate continues to be the gold standard in the treatment of rheumatoid arthritis and is widely utilized in other inflammatory diseases due to its proven efficacy and well-established safety profile [103]. Azathioprine and mycophenolate mofetil are preferred in diseases with systemic involvement, such as lupus with renal involvement, due to their systemic immunosuppressive effect [104]. In severe or refractory forms, cyclophosphamide, administered intravenously or orally, is considered an effective option, although associated with significant toxicity [105]. Choosing an appropriate corticosteroid-sparing therapy requires consideration of the specific pathology, disease severity, and the patient's comorbidities.

5.2 Biologics and small molecules in steroid-dependent diseases

The advent of biologic and small molecule therapies has revolutionized treatment for inflammatory and autoimmune conditions, offering a viable substitute for glucocorticoids in patients with severe or steroid-dependent disease.

TNF-α inhibitors, such as infliximab, adalimumab, and etanercept, have proven effective in treating rheumatoid arthritis, ankylosing spondylitis, and psoriasis, helping to reduce the need for prolonged glucocorticoid therapy [106]. In systemic lupus erythematosus, belimumab, a B-cell activating factor (BAFF) inhibitor, has been shown to control disease activity and facilitate gradual corticosteroid tapering [107].

Small molecules, particularly JAK inhibitors (e.g., tofacitinib and baricitinib), have recently expanded treatment options, offering effective oral therapies for rheumatoid arthritis and ulcerative colitis while reducing the need for corticosteroids [108].

In ANCA-positive vasculitis, the use of rituximab has allowed for remission and reduced glucocorticoid requirements, and is recommended in current guidelines as induction and maintenance therapy [109].

5.3 Role of lifestyle and non-pharmacologic interventions

Nonpharmacological interventions and lifestyle changes are an essential complementary element in reducing glucocorticoid dependence and improving the long-term prognosis of patients.

Regular physical activity, adapted to functional capacity, has beneficial effects on musculoskeletal status, contributing to the prevention of corticosteroid-induced osteoporosis and the maintenance of muscle mass [110]. Physical exercise can also improve fatigue and joint stiffness in rheumatic diseases [111].

Maintaining a diet rich in calcium and vitamin D is essential to reduce the risk of metabolic consequences such as osteoporosis and weight gain related to glucocorticoid therapy [77]. In addition, psychological counseling and cognitive-behavioral interventions can help reduce stress and improve adherence to treatment, factors that indirectly influence disease activity [112].

An integrated management approach includes smoking cessation and control of cardiovascular risk factors, given that patients with autoimmune disorders have an inherently higher cardiovascular risk, amplified by chronic glucocorticoid therapy [113].

6. Emerging insights and future directions

Glucocorticoids have remained a cornerstone of treatment for inflammatory and autoimmune disorders over the past several decades. However, differences in treatment response, cumulative adverse effects, and the lack of dependable predictive markers have spurred research into personalized therapy and the design of safer therapeutic agents. This has led to three main areas of focus: biomarker identification, personalized medicine applications, and the development of selective glucocorticoid receptor modulators (SEGRMs).

6.1 Biomarkers of corticosteroid responsiveness

A major limitation in glucocorticoid management is the lack of validated biomarkers capable of forecasting treatment response and side-effect risk. Emerging studies suggest that transcriptomic, genetic, and epigenetic factors could serve as tools for tailoring therapy to individual patients [19, 114].

Higher levels of NR3C1 gene expression, responsible for encoding the glucocorticoid receptor, are associated with better treatment outcomes in patients with RA and SLE [89]. Furthermore, genetic variations in enzymes involved in glucocorticoid metabolism, such as 11β-HSD1 and 11β-HSD2, can affect local corticosteroid activation and tissue responsiveness, with important clinical implications [40, 115].

The identification of reliable biomarkers could enable early adjustment of therapeutic strategies and limit unnecessary corticosteroid exposure, thereby reducing the risk of adverse effects.

6.2 Personalized medicine approaches

In the era of personalized medicine, integrating a patient's genetic, epigenetic, and phenotypic profile is increasingly critical for guiding glucocorticoid therapy. Next-generation sequencing and multiomics analyses provide deeper insights into the heterogeneity of glucocorticoid responses [116].

For example, in rheumatological diseases, subtyping patients based on gene expression signatures has proven useful in predicting therapeutic response and in the early selection of alternative strategies, such as biologics or small molecules [117]. At the same time, traditional clinical factors, such as disease severity, comorbidities, and cardiovascular risk, are integrated into personalized therapeutic decisions [118].

Personalized approaches have the potential to reduce glucocorticoid dependence, prevent adverse effects, and optimize patients' quality of life.

6.3 Novel glucocorticoid receptor modulators (SEGRMs)

An area of growing interest is the creation of Selective Glucocorticoid Receptor Modulators (SEGRMs), intended to preserve glucocorticoids' anti-inflammatory effects and reduce associated metabolic and adverse consequences [119].

SEGRMs act by promoting specific anti-inflammatory signaling pathways, with minimal inhibition of essential metabolic functions, such as bone or glycemic metabolism. Preclinical studies have demonstrated that these compounds can maintain anti-inflammatory efficacy in models of arthritis or systemic inflammatory diseases, with a significant reduction in associated adverse effects [120, 121].

A promising example is AZD9567, a SEGRM evaluated in early clinical trials, which demonstrated anti-inflammatory effects comparable to prednisone while exerting markedly less impact on the hypothalamic-pituitary-adrenal axis and bone metabolism [122].

The development and validation of SEGRMs could mark a revolutionary milestone in the treatment of inflammatory diseases, offering safer and better tolerated long-term therapeutic options.

7. Conclusions

Advances in our understanding of the molecular and cellular mechanisms underlying glucocorticoid responses provide new opportunities to optimize the treatment of inflammatory diseases. The identification of specific biomarkers and their integration into personalized medicine enables therapy to be tailored to individual patient needs, thereby minimizing adverse effects. The development of selective glucocorticoid receptor modulators offers a promising avenue for achieving effective treatment with an improved safety profile. Future research in this area is expected to enhance patient quality of life and reduce the long-term risks associated with corticosteroid therapy. In parallel, the adoption of complementary therapies, such as corticosteroid-sparing agents and biological therapies, contributes to reducing the required doses of glucocorticoids, thus minimizing toxicity. The future of glucocorticoid treatment looks promising, especially due to new research directions targeting response biomarkers, personalized medicine and selective glucocorticoid receptor modulators, capable of providing increased efficacy with reduced side effects.

Conflict of interest

The author declares no conflict of interest.

Author details

Cristina Criveanu
University of Medicine and Pharmacy of Craiova, Craiova, Romania

*Address all correspondence to: cristina.criveanu@yahoo.com

References

[1] Osler W, Mccrae T. The Principles and Practice of Medicine. 9th ed. New York: Appleton & Co; 1920. p. 859

[2] Burns CM. The history of cortisone discovery and development. Rheumatic Diseases Clinics of North America. 2016;**42**(1):1-14, vii. DOI: 10.1016/j.rdc.2015.08.001

[3] Benedek TG. Tadeus Reichstein, 1950. In: Fox DM, Meldrum M, Rezak I, editors. Nobel Laureates in Medicine or Physiology. New York: Garland Publishing; 1990. pp. 457-462

[4] Mason HL, Myers CS, Kendall EC. The chemistry of cystalline substances isolated from the suprarenal gland. The Journal of Biological Chemistry. 1936;**114**:613-631

[5] Hench PS, Kendall EC, Slocumb CH, et al. The effect of a hormone of the adrenal cortex (17-hydroxy-11-dehydrocorticosterone: Compound E) and of pituitary adrenocorticotropic hormone on rheumatoid arthritis. Preliminary report. Proceedings of the Staff Meetings of the Mayo Clinic. 1949;**24**:181-197

[6] Benedek TG. History of the development of corticosteroid therapy. Clinical and Experimental Rheumatology. 2011;**29**(5 Suppl. 68): 5-12. Epub 2011 Oct 21

[7] Nicolaides NC, Chrousos G, Kino T. Glucocorticoid Receptor. In: Feingold KR, Ahmed SF, Anawalt B, et al., editors. Endotext [Internet]. South Dartmouth (MA): MDText.com, Inc.; 2000. Available from: https://www.ncbi.nlm.nih.gov/books/NBK279171/ [Accessed: November 21, 2020]

[8] Lu NZ, Cidlowski JA. The origin and functions of multiple human glucocorticoid receptor isoforms. Annals of the New York Academy of Sciences. 2004;**1024**:102-123. DOI: 10.1196/annals.1321.008

[9] Oakley RH, Sar M, Cidlowski JA. The human glucocorticoid receptor beta isoform. Expression, biochemical properties, and putative function. The Journal of Biological Chemistry. 1996;**271**:9550-9559. DOI: 10.1074/jbc.271.16.9550

[10] Oakley RH, Jewell CM, Yudt MR, Bofetiado DM, Cidlowski JA. The dominant negative activity of the human glucocorticoid receptor β isoform specificity and mechanisms of action. The Journal of Biological Chemistry. 1999;**274**:27857-27866. DOI: 10.1074/jbc.274.39.27857

[11] Charmandari E, Chrousos GP, Ichijo T, Bhattacharyya N, Vottero A, Souvatzoglou E, et al. The human glucocorticoid receptor (hGR) β isoform suppresses the transcriptional activity of hGRα by interfering with formation of active coactivator complexes. Molecular Endocrinology. 2005;**19**:52-64. DOI: 10.1210/me.2004-0112

[12] Spiga F, Walker JJ, Terry JR, Lightman SL. HPA axis-rhythms. Comprehensive Physiology. 2014;**4**:1273-1298. DOI: 10.1002/cphy.c140003

[13] Malkoski SP, Dorin RI. Composite glucocorticoid regulation at a functionally defined negative glucocorticoid response element of the human corticotropin-releasing hormone gene. Molecular Endocrinology. 1999;**13**:1629-1644. DOI: 10.1210/mend.13.10.0351

[14] Drouin J, Lin S, Nemer M. Glucocorticoid repression of pro-opiomelanocortin gene transcription. Journal of Steroid Biochemistry. 1989;**34**:63-69. DOI: 10.1016/0022-4731(89)90066-6

[15] De Kloet R, Vreugdenhil E, Oitzl MS, Joëls M. Brain corticosteroid receptor balance in health and disease. Endocrine Reviews. 1998;**19**:269-301. DOI: 10.1210/er.19.3.269

[16] Martens C, Bilodeau S, Maira M, Gauthier Y, Drouin J. Protein-protein interactions and transcriptional antagonism between the subfamily of NGFI-B/Nur77 orphan nuclear receptors and glucocorticoid receptor. Molecular Endocrinology. 2005;**19**:885-897. DOI: 10.1210/me.2004-0333

[17] Bilodeau S, Vallette-Kasic S, Gauthier Y, Figarella-Branger D, Brue T, Berthelet F, et al. Role of Brg1 and HDAC2 in GR trans-repression of the pituitary POMC gene and misexpression in Cushing disease. Genes & Development. 2006;**20**:2871-2886. DOI: 10.1101/gad.1444606

[18] Oakley RH, Cidlowski JA. The biology of the glucocorticoid receptor: New signaling mechanisms in health and disease. Journal of Allergy and Clinical Immunology. 2013;**132**(5):1033-1044. DOI: 10.1016/j.jaci.2013.09.007

[19] Barnes PJ. Mechanisms and resistance in glucocorticoid control of inflammation. Journal of Steroid Biochemistry and Molecular Biology. 2010;**120**(2-3):76-85. DOI: 10.1016/j.jsbmb.2010.02.018

[20] Newton R, Holden NS. Separating transrepression and transactivation: A distressing divorce for the glucocorticoid receptor? Molecular Pharmacology. 2007;**72**(4):799-809. DOI: 10.1124/mol.107.038141

[21] Almawi WY, Melemedjian OK. Negative regulation of nuclear factor-κB activation and function by glucocorticoids. Journal of Molecular Endocrinology. 2002;**28**(2):69-78. DOI: 10.1677/jme.0.0280069

[22] Di S, Malcher-Lopes R, Halmos K, Tasker JG. Nongenomic glucocorticoid inhibition via endocannabinoid release in the hypothalamus: A fast feedback mechanism. The Journal of Neuroscience. 2003;**23**:4850-4857. DOI: 10.1523/JNEUROSCI.23-12-04850.2003

[23] Di S, Maxson MM, Franco A, Tasker JG. Glucocorticoids regulate glutamate and GABA synapse-specific retrograde transmission via divergent nongenomic signaling pathways. The Journal of Neuroscience. 2009;**29**:393-401. DOI: 10.1523/JNEUROSCI.4546-08.2009

[24] Buttgereit F et al. Standard and nonstandard effects of glucocorticoids: A review of their mechanisms of action in rheumatic diseases. Arthritis & Rheumatism. 1999;**42**(4):761-772. DOI: 10.1002/1529-0131(199904)42:4<761::AID-ANR15>3.0.CO;2-M

[25] Czock D, Keller F, Rasche FM, Häussler U. Pharmacokinetics and pharmacodynamics of systemically administered glucocorticoids. Clinical Pharmacokinetics. 2005;**44**(1):61-98. DOI: 10.2165/00003088-200544010-00003

[26] Schimmer BP, Funder JW. ACTH, adrenal steroids, and pharmacology of the adrenal cortex. In: Brunton LL, Hilal-Dandan R, Knollmann BC, editors. Goodman & Gilman's: The Pharmacological Basis of Therapeutics. 13th ed. New York: McGraw-Hill Education; 2017. pp. 747-773

[27] Derendorf H, Hochhaus G, Meibohm B, Barth J, Möllmann H.

Pharmacokinetics and pharmacodynamics of glucocorticoid preparations. Journal of Clinical Pharmacology. 1993;**33**(2):115-123

[28] Buttgereit F, Burmester GR, Straub RH. Exogenous and endogenous glucocorticoids in rheumatic diseases. Arthritis & Rheumatism. 2005;**52**(10):3139-3150

[29] Hämäläinen M, Moilanen E, Korhonen R. Pharmacokinetics of glucocorticoids: Key therapeutic and toxicological considerations. European Journal of Clinical Pharmacology. 2021;**77**:1-13

[30] Rose JQ, Yates CR, Meibohm B. Pharmacokinetics and pharmacodynamics of corticosteroids in health and disease. Clinical Pharmacokinetics. 2001;**40**(6):385-404

[31] Confavreux C, Aimard G, Devic M. Corticosteroids in the treatment of multiple sclerosis: Clinical pharmacology and therapeutic applications. Drugs. 1990;**39**(5):661-682

[32] Miller R, Greenberg DA. Clinical Pharmacology. New York: McGraw-Hill Education; 2019

[33] Rhen T, Cidlowski JA. Antiinflammatory action of glucocorticoids—New mechanisms for old drugs. The New England Journal of Medicine. 2005;**353**(16):1711-1723

[34] Hollander JL, Brown EM, Jessar RA. Hydrocortisone and cortisone injected into arthritic joints. Comparative effects of and use of hydrocortisone as a local antiarthritic agent. JAMA. 1951;**147**:1629-1635

[35] Bailey E, Greaves MS, Murphy D, West HF. Corticosteroid metabolism and rheumatoid arthritis. Annals of the Rheumatic Diseases. 1966;**25**:516-524

[36] Murphy D, West HF. Catabolism and interconversion of cortisol and cortisone in human synovial tissue in vitro. Annals of the Rheumatic Diseases. 1969;**28**:637-643

[37] Wilson H, Fairbanks R, Scialabba D, McEwen C, Ziff M. Metabolites of hydrocortisone and cortisone in synovial fluid in rheumatoid arthritis. The Journal of Clinical Endocrinology and Metabolism. 1956;**16**:86-113

[38] Olsen N, Sokka T, Seehorn CL, Kraft B, Maas K, Moore J, et al. A gene expression signature for recent onset rheumatoid arthritis in peripheral blood mononuclear cells. Annals of the Rheumatic Diseases. 2004;**63**:1387-1392

[39] Schmidt M, Weidler C, Naumann H, Anders S, Scholmerich J, Straub RH. Reduced capacity for the reactivation of glucocorticoids in rheumatoid arthritis synovial cells: Possible role of the sympathetic nervous system? Arthritis and Rheumatism. 2005;**52**:1711-1720

[40] Hardy R, Rabbitt EH, Filer A, Emery P, Hewison M, Stewart PM, et al. Local and systemic glucocorticoid metabolism in inflammatory arthritis. Annals of the Rheumatic Diseases. 2008;**67**(9):1204-1210

[41] Hazes JM, Verstappen SM, van der Maas A, Stalman W, Landewe RB, van der Heijde DM, et al. Individual patient data meta-analysis on continued use of glucocorticoids after their initiation as bridging therapy in patients with rheumatoid arthritis. Annals of the Rheumatic Diseases. 2021;**80**(3):355-363

[42] Fanouriakis A, Kostopoulou M, Alunno A, Aringer M, Bajema I, Boletis J, et al. 2019 update of the EULAR recommendations for the management of systemic lupus erythematosus.

Annals of the Rheumatic Diseases. 2019;**78**(6):736-745

[43] Hahn BH, McMahon MA, Wilkinson A, Wallace WD, Daikh DI, Fitzgerald JD, et al. American College of Rheumatology guidelines for screening, treatment, and management of lupus nephritis. Arthritis Care & Research (Hoboken). 2012;**64**(6):797-808

[44] Doria A, Gatto M, Zen M, Iaccarino L, Punzi L. Optimizing glucocorticoid use in systemic lupus erythematosus. Current Opinion in Rheumatology. 2017;**29**(6):650-656

[45] Gordon PA, Winer JB. Glucocorticoids in connective tissue diseases. Practical Neurology. 2012;**12**(6):356-361

[46] Jennette JC, Falk RJ, Bacon PA, Basu N, Cid MC, Ferrario F, et al. 2012 revised international Chapel Hill consensus conference nomenclature of vasculitides. Arthritis and Rheumatism. 2013;**65**(1):1-11

[47] Mukhtyar C, Guillevin L, Cid MC, Dasgupta B, de Groot K, Gross W, et al. EULAR recommendations for the management of primary small and medium vessel vasculitis. Annals of the Rheumatic Diseases. 2009;**68**(3):310-317

[48] Hellmich B, Agueda A, Monti S, Buttgereit F, de Boysson H, Brouwer E, et al. 2023 EULAR recommendations for the management of large vessel vasculitis. Annals of the Rheumatic Diseases. 2023;**82**(1):19-30

[49] Mecoli CA, Adler BL, Lee I, Christopher-Stine L. Glucocorticoid use in idiopathic inflammatory myopathies: Indications, dosing, and management of side effects. Current Rheumatology Reports. 2018;**20**(9):52

[50] Allenbach Y, Benveniste O, Stenzel W, Boyer O. Immune-mediated necrotizing myopathies: Clinical features and pathogenesis. Nature Reviews Rheumatology. 2020;**16**(12):689-701

[51] FitzGerald JD, Dalbeth N, Mikuls TR, et al. 2020 American College of Rheumatology Guideline for the Management of Gout. Arthritis Care & Research (Hoboken). 2020;**72**(6):744-760

[52] Khanna D, Khanna PP, Fitzgerald JD, et al. 2012 American College of Rheumatology guidelines for management of gout. Part 1: Systematic nonpharmacologic and pharmacologic therapeutic approaches to hyperuricemia. Arthritis Care & Research (Hoboken). 2012;**64**(10):1431-1446

[53] Schlesinger N, Lipsky PE. Glucocorticoids in the management of gout: A review of the evidence. Seminars in Arthritis and Rheumatism. 2020;**50**(1):31-38

[54] Abhishek A, Doherty M. Epidemiology and outcome of calcium pyrophosphate crystal deposition disease. Rheumatic Diseases Clinics of North America. 2014;**40**(2):177-191

[55] Khanna D, Khanna PP, Fitzgerald JD, et al. 2012 American College of Rheumatology guidelines for management of gout. Arthritis Care & Research (Hoboken). 2012;**64**(10):1431-1446

[56] Man CY, Cheung IT, Cameron PA, Rainer TH. Comparison of prednisolone and naproxen in the treatment of acute gout. A double-blind, randomized, controlled trial. Annals of Internal Medicine. 2007;**147**(10):653-660

[57] Goodman SM, Bykerk VP. Local corticosteroid injections: Current

practice and future directions. Nature Reviews Rheumatology. 2019;**15**(7):391-403

[58] Habib GS. Systemic effects of intra-articular corticosteroids. Clinical Rheumatology. 2009;**28**(7):749-756

[59] Weitoft T, Uddenfeldt P. Importance of synovial fluid aspiration when injecting intra-articular corticosteroids. Annals of the Rheumatic Diseases. 2000;**59**(11):975-977

[60] Kim SH, Ha CW, Park YB, et al. Intra-articular corticosteroid injection for knee osteoarthritis: A critical literature review. The American Journal of Sports Medicine. 2021;**49**(10):2817-2829

[61] McAlindon TE, LaValley MP, Harvey WF, et al. Effect of intra-articular triamcinolone vs saline on knee cartilage volume and pain in patients with knee osteoarthritis: A randomized clinical trial. Journal of the American Medical Association. 2017;**317**(19):1967-1975

[62] Sytsma TT, Greenlund LK, Greenlund LS. Joint infection after intra-articular steroid injection: A systematic review. Seminars in Arthritis and Rheumatism. 2018;**48**(4):638-643

[63] Gulliford MC, Charlton J, Latinovic R. Risk of diabetes associated with prescribed glucocorticoids in a large population. Diabetes Care. 2006;**29**(12):2728-2729

[64] Fardet L, Petersen I, Nazareth I. Risk of diabetes mellitus associated with long-term oral glucocorticoid use: A cohort study. BMJ Open. 2012;**2**(3):e000533

[65] van Raalte DH, Diamant M. Steroid diabetes: From mechanism to treatment? The Netherlands Journal of Medicine. 2014;**72**(2):62-72

[66] Cushing H. The basophil adenomas of the pituitary body and their clinical manifestations. Bulletin of the Johns Hopkins Hospital. 1932;**50**:137-195

[67] Compston J. Glucocorticoid-induced osteoporosis: An update. Endocrine. 2018;**61**(1):7-16

[68] van Staa TP, Leufkens HG, Cooper C. The epidemiology of corticosteroid-induced osteoporosis: A meta-analysis. Osteoporosis International. 2002;**13**(10):777-787

[69] Charmandari E, Nicolaides NC, Chrousos GP. Adrenal insufficiency. Lancet. 2014;**383**(9935):2152-2167

[70] Canalis E, Mazziotti G, Giustina A, Bilezikian JP. Glucocorticoid-induced osteoporosis: Pathophysiology and therapy. Osteoporosis International. 2007;**18**(10):1319-1328

[71] Weinstein RS. Clinical practice: Glucocorticoid-induced bone disease. The New England Journal of Medicine. 2011;**365**(1):62-70

[72] O'Brien CA, Jia D, Plotkin LI, et al. Glucocorticoids act directly on osteoblasts and osteocytes to induce their apoptosis and reduce bone formation. Endocrinology. 2004;**145**(4):1835-1841

[73] Hofbauer LC, Rauner M. Minireview: Molecular understanding of bone loss in glucocorticoid-induced osteoporosis. Molecular Endocrinology. 2009;**23**(11):1529-1538

[74] Pereira RM, Freire de Carvalho J. Glucocorticoid-induced myopathy. Journal of Clinical Rheumatology. 2011;**17**(6):287-290

[75] Saag KG, Emkey R, Schnitzer TJ, et al. Alendronate for the prevention and treatment of glucocorticoid-induced

osteoporosis. The New England Journal of Medicine. 1998;**339**(5):292-299

[76] van Staa TP, Geusens P, Pols HA, et al. A simple clinical risk score for osteoporosis in men and women: The Rotterdam study. The Journal of Rheumatology. 2006;**33**(5):1022-1030

[77] Buckley L, Humphrey MB. Glucocorticoid-induced osteoporosis. The New England Journal of Medicine. 2018;**379**(26):2547-2556

[78] Grossman JM, Gordon R, Ranganath VK, et al. American College of Rheumatology 2010 recommendations for the prevention and treatment of glucocorticoid-induced osteoporosis. Arthritis Care and Research. 2010;**62**(11):1515-1526

[79] Walker BR. Glucocorticoids and cardiovascular disease. European Journal of Endocrinology. 2007;**157**(5):545-559

[80] Fardet L, Petersen I, Nazareth I. Risk of cardiovascular events in people prescribed glucocorticoids with iatrogenic Cushing's syndrome: Cohort study. BMJ. 2012;**345**:e4928

[81] Whitworth JA. Mechanisms of glucocorticoid-induced hypertension. Kidney International. 1987;**31**(3):1213-1223

[82] Wei L, MacDonald TM, Walker BR. Taking glucocorticoids by prescription is associated with subsequent cardiovascular disease. Annals of Internal Medicine. 2004;**141**(10):764-770

[83] Souverein PC, Berard A, Van Staa TP, et al. Use of oral glucocorticoids and risk of cardiovascular and cerebrovascular disease in a population based case-control study. Heart. 2004;**90**(8):859-865

[84] Warrington TP, Bostwick JM. Psychiatric adverse effects of corticosteroids. Mayo Clinic Proceedings. 2006;**81**(10):1361-1367

[85] Brown ES, Chandler PA. Mood and cognitive changes during systemic corticosteroid therapy. Primary Care Companion to the Journal of Clinical Psychiatry. 2001;**3**(1):17-21

[86] Lupien SJ, McEwen BS, Gunnar MR, Heim C. Effects of stress throughout the lifespan on the brain, behaviour and cognition. Nature Reviews. Neuroscience. 2009;**10**(6):434-445

[87] Brown ES, Suppes T. Mood symptoms during corticosteroid therapy: A review. Harvard Review of Psychiatry. 1998;**5**(5):239-246

[88] Ciriaco M, Ventrice P, Russo G, et al. Corticosteroid-related central nervous system side effects. Journal of Pharmacology and Pharmacotherapeutics. 2013;**4**(Suppl. 1):S94-S98

[89] Schäcke H, Döcke WD, Asadullah K. Mechanisms involved in the side effects of glucocorticoids. Pharmacology & Therapeutics. 2002;**96**(1):23-43

[90] Doran MF, Crowson CS, Pond GR, O'Fallon WM, Gabriel SE. Frequency of infection in patients with rheumatoid arthritis compared with controls: A population-based study. Arthritis and Rheumatism. 2002;**46**(9):2287-2293

[91] Dixon WG, Suissa S, Hudson M. The association between systemic glucocorticoid therapy and the risk of infection in patients with rheumatoid arthritis: Systematic review and meta-analyses. Arthritis Research & Therapy. 2011;**13**(4):R139

[92] van Staa TP, Leufkens HG, Abenhaim L, Zhang B, Cooper C. Use of oral corticosteroids and risk of fractures.

Journal of Bone and Mineral Research. 2000;**15**(6):993-1000

[93] Winthrop KL. The emerging safety profile of JAK inhibitors in rheumatic disease. Nature Reviews Rheumatology. 2017;**13**(4):234-243

[94] Jick SS, Lieberman ES, Rahman MU, Choi HK. Glucocorticoid use, other associated factors, and the risk of tuberculosis. Arthritis and Rheumatism. 2006;**55**(1):19-26

[95] Gianfrancesco M, Hyrich KL, Al-Adely S, et al. Characteristics associated with hospitalisation for COVID-19 in people with rheumatic disease: Data from the COVID-19 global rheumatology Alliance physician-reported registry. Annals of the Rheumatic Diseases. 2020;**79**(7):859-866

[96] Fardet L, Petersen I, Nazareth I. Risk of infections with glucocorticoids: A meta-analysis of observational studies. JAMA Internal Medicine. 2016;**176**(9):1266-1276

[97] Cain DW, Cidlowski JA. Immune regulation by glucocorticoids. Nature Reviews. Immunology. 2017;**17**(4):233-247

[98] Moutsopoulos HM, Fragoulis GE, Sfikakis PP. Vaccination in autoimmune rheumatic disease. Current Opinion in Rheumatology. 2022;**34**(3):197-205

[99] Furer V, Rondaan C, Heijstek MW, et al. 2019 update of EULAR recommendations for vaccination in adult patients with autoimmune inflammatory rheumatic diseases. Annals of the Rheumatic Diseases. 2020;**79**(1):39-52

[100] Yale SH, Limper AH. Pneumocystis carinii pneumonia in patients without acquired immunodeficiency syndrome: Associated illnesses and prior corticosteroid therapy. Mayo Clinic Proceedings. 1996;**71**(1):5-13

[101] van Vollenhoven RF. Treatment of rheumatoid arthritis: State of the art 2009. Nature Reviews Rheumatology. 2009;**5**(10):531-541

[102] Hahn BH, McMahon MA, Wilkinson A, et al. American College of Rheumatology guidelines for screening, treatment, and management of lupus nephritis. Arthritis Care and Research. 2012;**64**(6):797-808

[103] Smolen JS, Landewé R, Bijlsma J, et al. EULAR recommendations for the management of rheumatoid arthritis. Annals of the Rheumatic Diseases. 2020;**79**(6):685-699

[104] Parikh SV, Almaani S, Brodsky S, Rovin BH. Update on lupus nephritis. Clinical Journal of the American Society of Nephrology. 2020;**15**(5):673-682

[105] Jayne D, Rasmussen N, Andrassy K, et al. A randomized trial of maintenance therapy for vasculitis associated with ANCA. The New England Journal of Medicine. 2003;**349**(1):36-44

[106] Singh JA, Saag KG, Bridges SL Jr, et al. 2015 American College of Rheumatology guideline for the treatment of rheumatoid arthritis. Arthritis & Rhematology. 2016;**68**(1):1-26

[107] Furie R, Rovin BH, Houssiau F, et al. Two-year, randomized, controlled trial of belimumab in lupus nephritis. The New England Journal of Medicine. 2020;**383**(12):1117-1128

[108] McInnes IB, Byers NL, Higgs RE, et al. Comparison of baricitinib, tofacitinib, and upadacitinib in rheumatoid arthritis: A systematic

review. The Lancet Rheumatology. 2021;**3**(7):e498-e507

[109] Jones RB, Furuta S, Tervaert JW, et al. Rituximab versus cyclophosphamide in ANCA-associated vasculitis: A meta-analysis. Annals of the Rheumatic Diseases. 2019;**78**(3):384-391

[110] Lemmey AB, Williams SL, Marcora SM, et al. Resistance exercise improves muscle strength and physical function in rheumatoid arthritis patients. Arthritis Care and Research. 2009;**61**(12):1726-1734

[111] Baillet A, Vaillant M, Guinot M, et al. Efficacy of cardiorespiratory aerobic exercise in rheumatoid arthritis: Meta-analysis. Arthritis Care and Research. 2010;**62**(7):984-992

[112] Matcham F, Rayner L, Steer S, Hotopf M. The prevalence of depression in rheumatoid arthritis: A systematic review. Rheumatology (Oxford, England). 2013;**52**(12):2136-2148

[113] Aviña-Zubieta JA, Choi HK, Sadatsafavi M, et al. Risk of cardiovascular mortality in patients with rheumatoid arthritis: A meta-analysis. Arthritis and Rheumatism. 2008;**59**(12):1690-1697

[114] Coutinho AE, Chapman KE. The anti-inflammatory and immunosuppressive effects of glucocorticoids. Clinical and Experimental Immunology. 2011;**158**(3):256-265

[115] Tiganescu A, Hupe M, Danilenko M, et al. 11β-HSD1 deficiency protects against age-related skin structure and function defects. The Journal of Clinical Investigation. 2013;**123**(7):3051-3060

[116] Dennis G Jr, Holweg CT, Kummerfeld SK, et al. Synovial phenotypes in rheumatoid arthritis correlate with response to biologic therapeutics. Arthritis Research & Therapy. 2014;**16**(2):R90

[117] Humby F, Lewis M, Ramamoorthi N, et al. Synovial tissue phenotypes predict response to biologic agents in rheumatoid arthritis. Nature Communications. 2019;**10**(1):2166

[118] Smolen JS, Aletaha D, McInnes IB. Rheumatoid arthritis. Lancet. 2016;**388**(10055):2023-2038

[119] Schäcke H, Berger M, Rehwinkel H, Asadullah K. Selective glucocorticoid receptor agonists (SEGRAs): Novel ligands with an improved therapeutic index. Molecular and Cellular Endocrinology. 2007;**275**(1-2):109-117

[120] Sundahl N, Bridelance J, Libert C, et al. Selective glucocorticoid receptor modulation: New directions with non-steroidal scaffolds. Pharmacology & Therapeutics. 2015;**152**:28-41

[121] Webster JC, Oakley RH, Jewell CM, et al. Proinflammatory cytokines regulate human glucocorticoid receptor gene expression and lead to glucocorticoid resistance. Journal of Immunology. 2001;**167**(12):7184-7192

[122] Högberg C, Svensson D, Delbro DS, et al. AZD9567, a novel selective glucocorticoid receptor modulator with anti-inflammatory efficacy and an improved side effect profile. Scientific Reports. 2021;**11**(1):24548